Regain Your Brain

EPISODE TRANSCRIPTS

Exclusive Interviews
Conducted by Peggy Sarlin

Regain Your Brain Episode Transcripts
By Peggy Sarlin

Published by Online Publishing & Marketing, LLC

IMPORTANT CAUTION:

By reading these interview transcripts, you are demonstrating an interest in maintaining good and vigorous health. These interviews suggest ways you can do that but – as with anything in medicine – there are no guarantees. You must consult privately with medical advisors to assess whether the suggestions in these interviews are appropriate for you – or you must accept full responsibility if you decide not to do so. Neither Peggy Sarlin nor the doctors and other authorities she spoke with in these interviews meant their comments to be personal medical advice for any particular individual.

The views expressed herein are those of the doctors and experts who voice them and not necessarily those of Peggy Sarlin or the editors and publishers. Peggy Sarlin is a writer, not a physician, doctor or professional health caregiver and her comments herein are not intended as personal medical advice.

The author, editors and publishers of this volume are not responsible for any adverse effects or results from the use of any of the suggestions, preparations or procedures the report describes. As with any medical treatment, the results described in this report will vary from one person to another. The author, editors and publishers believe the information in this volume is accurate but they cannot guarantee its accuracy.

ISBN 978-1-5323-1688-3

Printed in the United States of America

ABOUT THE AUTHOR

Peggy Sarlin is a freelance writer with a special interest in health and wellness. She wrote the first book to investigate alternative remedies for Alzheimer's disease. Published in 2012, *Awakening from Alzheimer's: How 9 Maverick Doctors Are Reversing Alzheimer's, Dementia, and Memory Loss* has informed thousands of people about safe natural options for cognitive health. Over the past several years, Peggy has journeyed tirelessly across the U.S., interviewing the world's most renowned doctors on the frontlines of the war against Alzheimer's and dementia. She shared their stories with the public in two free online video series, *Awakening from Alzheimer's: The Event*, and *Regain Your Brain*.

Contents

Pilot Episode

You're Not Stuck With the Brain You've Got (But You Have to Have a Plan)

DANIEL AMEN: Well, the message of my life is: You're not stuck with the brain you have. You can make it better, even if you've been bad to it. You just have to put it in a healing environment.

CUT TO:

DAVID PERLMUTTER: The notion that the brain can grow new brain cells, for example, is brand new. That was only published in 1998. Before that, there had been this huge rejection of the notion that humans had a second chance.

And only in the past few years have we understood not just that we have this opportunity to grow new brain cells, but that, in addition, we can enhance the process. These are brand-new cells. They are stem cells in the brain.

CUT TO:

DANIEL AMEN: It has the storage capacity of six million years of The Wall Street Journal, if you take care of it.

CUT TO:

NORMAN DOIDGE: In small parts of the brain, one can actually grow new cells, and it turns out that those small parts of the brain are actually relevant for Alzheimer's. Throughout the brain, through the rest of the brain, you can change the connectivity between the cells. You can grow new connections, or prune away various other connections to actually change the networks in the brain.

CUT TO:

DALE BREDESEN: As you know, your brain is important. And if that's not working, then it doesn't really matter if everything else is working, because if your brain's not working, you're in trouble.

CUT TO:

DALE BREDESEN: And that's the thing, that's the reason everyone should be coming in earlier and earlier – and preferably be on prevention, but if you've missed the prevention part, and you've started to have some symptoms, then come in and get on the program earlier. Get yourself evaluated so that you can turn this around quickly.

CUT TO:

DALE BREDESEN: But we have seen unprecedented improvements in many people with pre-Alzheimer's, so-called MCI or SCI, as well as those with Alzheimer's disease. And we're learning lessons, such as, some of the people that we thought were too late for the program have actually done quite well on the program."

CUT TO:

DANIEL AMEN: Just last week, a really well-known best-selling author came to see us two years ago, and her brain was really a mess, and she was a mess – problems with memory, and focus, and irritability, and not being able to get work done. And she's 46.

By doing all the things we asked her to do, when we did her two-year follow-up scan, we found she is dramatically better, and her brain is dramatically better. And she has Alzheimer's disease in her family. At her first scan, our reaction was, "Oh, you're headed to the dark place." Because we can tell decades before you have any symptoms. And the exciting thing is, she's not stuck with that brain. She's not stuck with that trajectory. You just have to be serious, and you have to have a plan.

CUT TO:

PEGGY SARLIN AND LEE EULER IN THE STUDIO:

PEGGY: You just have to have a plan. You're not stuck with the brain you've got, but you have to have a plan.

Hello, I'm Peggy Sarlin, the author of *Awakening from Alzheimer's*, and I'm your host for this very special event – Regain Your Brain. Today, I'm going to help you with *your* plan for protecting and saving your brain. As you can see from the clips we just played, no matter how old you are, no matter if you already have Alzheimer's disease or some other type of dementia... or if you're just starting to notice a little bit of memory loss and it bothers you... your brain can get better. You can recover and even come back stronger than ever.

And if you're young and healthy, you can boost your memory and cognitive ability to levels you never thought possible.

You're not stuck with the brain you've got, but you have to have a plan.

And you're in luck, because you're looking at the first of 12 episodes packed with the latest, cutting edge discoveries in brain health and neuroscience. You're going to meet doctors who are reversing Alzheimer's disease – not for every patient, but for many.

But there's more: Young, healthy people are using these tips to get sharper than they've ever been in their lives. They're using them to improve their performance in highly competitive jobs.

Now I'd like to introduce you to Lee Euler, the editor of the twice-weekly newsletter, Brain Health Breakthroughs. Lee is the publisher of my book and the producer of this video series.

LEE: Thanks, Peggy. I want to welcome all our viewers to Regain Your Brain, with a special "welcome back" to those who saw our first series, called Awakening from Alzheimer's.

So much has happened in just the two years since we filmed the first series. At that time, we were among the first to break the exciting news that Alzheimer's disease is now reversible. The big breakthroughs literally took place just before we interviewed the doctors.

PEGGY: That's right, Lee. Dr. Dale Bredesen, one of the doctors we just saw, had just published the first article in a major medical journal proving you can reverse Alzheimer's disease. And I talked to him and many other doctors who confirmed this amazing breakthrough.

LEE: Until that breakthrough, everyone – and I mean everyone – believed Alzheimer's disease is untreatable. Sad to say, most doctors will still tell you that – the same thing they told my family almost 20 years ago when my mother had Alzheimer's.

Revolutions in medical practice happen slowly. But things are moving. When we published our first series, fewer than a hundred doctors were putting the new discoveries to work. Today there are about a thousand doctors in the United States who have been trained in them and are treating patients.

PEGGY: In this series of video interviews, you're going to learn what they do, including things you can do at home, yourself, to start restoring normal memory to yourself or someone you love. Or to maximize your potential if you're healthy.

LEE: And things are moving so fast. Doctors know much more than they knew a couple of years ago, and we're going to bring it to you in this new series. Almost every day, a new breakthrough adds to our treasure trove of knowledge about what you can do to boost your memory and cognitive ability and even grow new brain cells, as some of the doctors at the beginning said.

PEGGY: That's right, Lee. Even people in advanced stages of this dreaded disease can recover some function. There are many, many documented cases, published in leading medical journals, where patients regained the ability to recognize their loved ones and perform the everyday functions of life that all of us take for granted, but that people lose in the late stages of dementia.

In fact, one of our big revelations in this series is that a total cure for dementia is in the works. I don't mean "treating" or "reversing" – I mean recovering all the functions of a young, healthy brain. This treatment is not quite here yet, but it will soon be in human trials, and things look very promising. It's really exciting.

LEE: I think this series will be the first to break this incredible news. But meanwhile, Peggy, when it comes to things our viewers can do right now, what strikes you as the most important single thing? Start our viewers off with the biggest takeaway from all the doctors and scientists you've interviewed for this new series.

PEGGY: Wow, Lee, that's a tough one. So much has happened, there are so many new discoveries. I would say the biggest takeaway is that brain plaques – the famous beta amyloid plaques – are NOT the cause of Alzheimer's disease. They're just a symptom.

LEE: That's big news, alright. All the medical research, all the drug company research has focused on getting rid of those plaques,

PEGGY: Right, and they've been barking up the wrong tree. There have been hundreds of trials of Alzheimer's drugs, and they've all failed. They don't do a bit of good. And almost all of them aimed at getting rid of beta amyloid plaques. And they didn't even make it to market. They did nothing to restore cognitive function. Let's take a look at what Dr. Bredesen has to say about that...

CUT TO:

DALE BREDESEN: What we found was actually diametrically opposed to the claim that when your brain makes amyloid, this is a bad thing for your brain, and this causes your brain to get damaged, and we want to get rid of that bad stuff.

What we found is, in fact, the opposite. Amyloid is a protective response that, in fact, we make in response to three different classes of pathogens and insults. And certainly, other groups, such as Dr. Moir and Dr. Tanzi from Harvard, have shown that there is an antimicrobial effect to amyloid, which fits into this whole, overall picture perfectly.

CUT TO:

PEGGY IN THE STUDIO:

PEGGY: So you see, the plaques are your body's effort to protect itself from an infection or toxin or another insult to the brain. Brain plaques are not the source of the problem, they're your body's effort to solve the problem. But let's get back to Dr. Bredesen...

CUT TO:

DALE BREDESEN: What happens is that we get exposed to a number of things during our lives, and as part of our protective response, we make the very stuff that the pathologist looks at and says, "Oh, you have Alzheimer's disease."

CUT TO:

MARY KAY ROSS: I think it's an effort on the body's part to protect you. Certainly, we think the plaques are a problem, and we can remove them or try to remove them. But you also want to understand why they're there, and you want to remove the insult that caused your body to make the plaques.

CUT TO:

PEGGY and LEE in the studio:

LEE: So the drugs are all about removing brain plaques, and that's why the drugs don't work.

PEGGY: Exactly right. If you go to a doctor with memory loss, you'll walk out the door with a prescription for a drug. There are four of them, Aricept, Namenda, Exelon or Razadyne. These drugs do just about nothing to help your brain function. And most doctors will tell you that's all they have and there's nothing else you can do.

LEE: What they really mean is, there's nothing more *they* can do. But we know better, thanks to the cutting-edge doctors you've interviewed. So you've told us what Alzheimer's isn't. Now tell us what it is.

PEGGY: Actually, Dr. Ross kind of hinted at the right approach in that last clip. We don't want to ask "what" it is, we want to ask "why." Why do we have this condition? The "what" is easy – you're losing your memory. Maybe you've just started having senior moments in the past year or two.

Or maybe you're farther down the path and you've got really serious memory loss. You may get confused, lose your sense of direction. And, yes, you may have brain plaques, even though half the people with dementia don't even have plaques.

LEE: Half the people with dementia don't have beta amyloid plaques?

PEGGY: Half the people with dementia don't have brain plaques. So what we've really got is a syndrome, a bunch of symptoms – memory loss, brain fog, maybe irritability, getting lost and confused. So let's ask "why." What got you to this place where you don't want to be?

And it turns out it isn't just one thing. It's not one disease or one big cause. There are many things that can get you to that place.

LEE: So Alzheimer's or dementia – whatever you want to call it – is not just one disease.

PEGGY: Right. And the doctors I talked to explain how you can diagnose what type of Alzheimer's you've got. They can help you find out how you got to this place where you don't want to be. In the next 12 days we're going to unpack all the things that cause memory loss and dementia, and what you can do about them. And some of them are really surprising.

LEE: Like what? Tell us.

PEGGY: Okay, this is another discovery that's just emerging. It's breaking news. As we mentioned earlier, toxins and infections – chronic infections – can be two big reasons for memory loss. And that was known a couple of years ago when we did our first series. But now it's coming out that a particular type of toxin may play a much bigger role than doctors thought: mold.

LEE: Mold? Like, in our homes, or what?

PEGGY: Yes, you're on the right track. Let's take a listen to Doctor Ross, an MD and the founder of the Institute for Personalized Medicine in Savannah, Georgia.

CUT TO:

MARY KAY ROSS: Well, I actually became a patient. I was exposed to mold in my home and became very ill. I developed respiratory problems. I developed thyroid problems, and I developed autoimmune disease. I had psoriatic arthritis, and in an effort to heal myself and find out, really, what my ailments were coming from and what I could do about them, I became involved in functional medicine.

I trained at the Institute for Functional Medicine, and it's become a big passion of mine. I've discovered, really, what a poor job traditional medicine does for chronic illness.

CUT TO:

PEGGY: This whole life change for you was a kind of random thing that happened to you because of exposure to mold. So tell us about that. What happens to people who are exposed to mold? What happens to their brains?

MARY KAY ROSS: It can have a very bad effect on your brain, obviously, and it can be a cause for Alzheimer's disease. Dr. Bredesen actually wrote a paper on inhalational Alzheimer's disease.

CUT TO:

PEGGY AND LEE IN THE STUDIO:

LEE: Inhalational Alzheimer's disease. That's a whole new concept. Let's pause it there for a second. You know, this has me wondering if mold can really be that big a factor in the Alzheimer's epidemic. Is this really something people need to be concerned about?

PEGGY: Good question. I asked Dr. Ross the very same thing. Here's what she said...

CUT TO:

MARY KAY ROSS: That's an interesting question, because when Dr. Bredesen first started doing his studying, he felt that this would probably be about 15% of the population.

PEGGY: One-five.

MARY KAY ROSS: And now we're realizing it's about 70%, and it may even be more. That's part of the study we're looking at. Because we're realizing that these markers, these inflammatory markers that we look at, which we thought would be in a very small group of people, are in a great many, and at this point we think it's about 70%.

PEGGY: Just to clarify, when we say 70%, it's not 70% of the population but 70% of the population presenting with Alzheimer's.

MARY KAY ROSS: Yes, that's correct.

PEGGY: So this may be the most significant factor.

MARY KAY ROSS: It may be a very large factor.

CUT TO:

PEGGY AND LEE IN THE STUDIO:

LEE: That's an amazing discovery if it holds up.

PEGGY: Yes, these are early days and these pioneering doctors are looking at mold and a host of other factors that undermine brain health and rob us of our memories. But the mold toxicity is looking like a hot area. Just listen to this real-life story...

CUT TO:

MARY KAY ROSS: Okay, I have a patient that's 52 years old, and she moved into a very old home. She was very healthy, a very well-educated engineer, and had a family of teenagers and college students. And suddenly she developed Alzheimer's.

Her family didn't see it coming initially, and then when they realized it, it was full-blown Alzheimer's. She had had an amyloid scan that was positive.

We did a lot of history-taking, and realized that she had had a lot of leaks in the house. It was very old. We tested the house, and the mold was through the roof in the house. So she had to move out of the house.

But she's actually getting better now. She's starting to drive with her children. She's actually going to the grocery with family members, actively shopping, putting her protocol together.

In the beginning, she couldn't do any of that. She's doing her brain studies every day. She works on brain exercises, and we're seeing great movement in the right direction.

CUT TO:

LEE AND PEGGY IN THE STUDIO:

LEE: That's quite a story. The mold problem is real.

PEGGY: It's absolutely real. My interview with Dr. Ross is airing on Day 5 of this series. She reveals the best medical way to remove mold toxins – they're called mycotoxins – the whole rundown on how to diagnose and treat the problem.

LEE: Yeah, I think people will want to tune in on Day 5 and hear about this new discovery. Are there are other microbes we need to be concerned about?

PEGGY: Yes. When someone seems to have Alzheimer's disease, it often happens that an underlying infection accounts for much of the problem. Lyme disease is a common cause, but let's let Dr. Daniel Amen give us the big picture...

CUT TO:

DANIEL AMEN: And infections are a major cause of dementia, and still not really well known.

PEGGY: I wanted to talk to you about that for a minute. Several doctors I've spoken to have really emphasized Lyme disease, this epidemic, which then can bring on cognitive problems. But you talk about a lot of other ones that aren't as well known, other viruses, parasites from your pet. You go into a whole bunch of things.

DANIEL AMEN: Toxoplasmosis, right.

PEGGY: Yes, yes. Epstein-Barr... Tell us about all these horrible things that we may not be thinking about.

DANIEL AMEN: I think the big issue is, if you have memory problems and they're not getting better with simple things, somebody should do an infectious disease panel to make sure you're not at war with some invader, like toxoplasmosis that comes from cat feces, or Lyme. Kris Kristofferson was diagnosed with Alzheimer's, and actually was found to have Lyme by one of our doctors, and was put on an antibiotic and hyperbaric oxygen. He got brought back, and he's touring again.

Herpes is another one. It's very common, and if you have genital herpes, or you have cold sores, it increases your risk of significant memory problems by 20%. And you know, that affects a third of the population.

CUT TO:

PAMELA WARTIAN SMITH: Lyme disease is huge. It can affect the brain and cognition. If we go back and treat that, then we may be able to retrieve some of the memory. Parasitic infections are a factor.

It is globalization of the world. People travel everywhere.

PEGGY: And they come back with parasites.

PAMELA WARTIAN SMITH: They do. And then the parasites can invade the brain as well. We give them an anti-parasitic agent, good bacteria... Those kinds of things are reversible causes of cognitive decline, commonly.

PEGGY: And I think it's fair to say that people can have more than one thing wrong with them at the same time. Again, the approach of coming at it from multiple angles.

CUT TO:

PEGGY AND LEE IN THE STUDIO:

LEE: This news about mold and infections is fascinating. But I have a question.

PEGGY: Okay...

LEE: In our first series the doctors put a huge emphasis on high blood sugar and insulin resistance as a cause of dementia. They said Alzheimer's disease is actually "Type 3 diabetes." Have molds and infections kind of superceded blood sugar?

PEGGY: Absolutely not. The evidence is stronger than ever that high blood sugar is a major cause of Alzheimer's disease. It's important for our viewers to understand this: Alzheimer's disease has multiple causes. I spoke with Dr. David Perlmutter, the best-selling author of *Grain Brain* and *Brain Maker,* about this whole topic of what causes Alzheimer's. Let's take a look...

CUT TO:

DAVID PERLMUTTER: The brain doesn't decline just because one thing is askew. Multiple things conspire to create an environment in which the brain then is unable to thrive. That said, you have to target as many of those entities as possible, if you're going to reverse Alzheimer's disease."

CUT TO:

MARY NEWPORT: And that is important in Alzheimer's disease because it is a type of diabetes of the brain. This may not be widely known. People know about plaques and amyls in the brain, but another very important aspect is that there's a problem with insulin resistance and insulin deficiency in the brain, very much like Type 2 diabetes, where there is a problem of getting glucose into brain cells in the areas that are affected by Alzheimer's.

CUT TO:

PAMELA WARTIAN SMITH: But your point is very well taken about diabetes, because sometimes people don't realize there are really three kinds of diabetes. There's Type I, where people don't make insulin at all. There's Type II, which is what 95% of Americans have who have diabetes. In Type II, they make insulin, but it doesn't work effectively in the body.

But now there's Type III diabetes, and that's Alzheimer's disease.

PEGGY: And this is a new way of thinking about Alzheimer's as well.

PAMELA WARTIAN SMITH: It is.

PEGGY: Which is that it's diabetes of the brain.

PAMELA WARTIAN SMITH: It is diabetes of the brain in many ways.

CUT TO:

DAVID PERLMUTTER: Individuals who do not develop Type 2 diabetes may have as much as a 50% reduction in the risk of Alzheimer's.

CUT TO:

PEGGY AND LEE BACK IN THE STUDIO:

LEE: That's Dr. Perlmutter saying diabetes increases your risk of Alzheimer's disease by 50%. So it's really important to manage your blood sugar.

PEGGY: High blood sugar is a huge risk factor. You have to deal with that or you're at risk of dementia. By the way, I want to tell our viewers that my interview with Dr. Perlmutter airs on Day 11 of this series. He's the best-selling author of *Grain Brain* and other books. You don't want to miss it because he has some blockbuster news and advice.

LEE: Give us a hint about what the blockbuster news is.

PEGGY: Well, he talks about the research that's going on worldwide and that's looking at questions like how do you boost the growth of new brain cells, and he mentioned a natural molecule that he says is fundamental to making this happen. But instead of me explaining it, let's take a sneak preview...

CUT TO:

DAVID PERLMUTTER: We know one chemical that happens to be really fundamental mechanistically in making this happen, allowing it to happen, is called BDNF. Now, that sounds a bit technical, but go with me on this.

PEGGY: Oh, I'm with you. Take me away on BDNF.

DAVID PERLMUTTER: BDNF is basically growth hormone for the brain. And when you have higher levels of BDNF, as research has demonstrated, you are resistant to getting Alzheimer's in the first place.

CUT TO:

DAVID PERLMUTTER: In fact, newer research correlates actual growth of the brain's memory center over one to two years in people with the highest level of BDNF, and that is revolutionary. You know, we all sort of accepted the notion that as we age, our brains will rust, as you mentioned, deteriorate, and shrink, and lose the ability to function.

We now understand this just isn't true. And it's taken a lot for people to embrace this as it relates to the brain, because we still tend to cling to this notion that we peak out around 18 years of age, and then after that it's "We're all on the skids." You know, you drink a beer, and that's 30,000 brain cells, and the next thing you know, you're in deep trouble when you're 50, or 60, or 80.

CUT TO:

DAVID PERLMUTTER: But that just isn't what our science is telling us anymore. What it's telling us is that when we amplify this chemical, BDNF, then we get a second chance.

CUT TO:

PEGGY AND LEE IN THE STUDIO:

LEE: A second chance. What a wonderful thing. It sounds to me like BDNF could be key to getting your brain back.

PEGGY: It's very exciting stuff. I can't begin to tell you how much I learned in talking to these doctors, and how much our viewers are going to discover in the next eleven days. It's life-changing news.

LEE: I've got to ask – Is there a way we can all boost our BDNF levels?

PEGGY: Absolutely. Tune in on Day 11 of this series. Dr. Perlmutter reveals the things we can do to boost BDNF levels. And the most powerful booster is something we can all do at home – and it's free.

LEE: That's incredible. I feel like just that one tip has the potential to change my life. Are there more like that?

PEGGY: Absolutely. Lots more. For example, several of the doctors I talked to really shined the light on hormones and hormone imbalances. Our first interview series talked about hormones, but in this new series, hormones are really front and center. Hormone deficiencies increase your risk of dementia. Let's listen to some highlights...

CUT TO:

DALE BREDESEN: And in fact, it's been shown by nice studies out of the Mayo Clinic that women who had early hysterectomies with oophorectomy, with loss of the ovaries, and who did not receive hormone replacement therapy, in fact doubled their likelihood of developing Alzheimer's later in life.

CUT TO:

PAMELA WARTIAN SMITH: For example, if we're looking at women or men, we do know that hormonal function has a lot to do with memory. For example, for men, testosterone literally equals memory. So if testosterone has started to decline, we want to measure it and replace it appropriately.

The same thing for women. Estrogen equals memory, so we measure and replace appropriately with the right kinds of estrogens. There's even a hormone of memory, and it's called pregnenolone. Have you ever heard of that hormone?

PEGGY: Well, I have. I read a lot about memory and the brain, but most people haven't. I think most people know estrogen and testosterone, but they don't know... okay. You pronounce it for me.

PAMELA WARTIAN SMITH: It's so funny to me that the hormone of memory would be hard to say – pregnenolone –

PEGGY: Pregnenolone.

PAMELA WARTIAN SMITH: And hard to spell. It's – to me, it's –

PEGGY: Hard to remember.

PAMELA WARTIAN SMITH: It is hard to remember.

PEGGY: It's hard to remember. But what does it do for us?

PAMELA WARTIAN SMITH: It's the mother hormone. It actually makes estrogen, progesterone, testosterone, DHEA and cortisol, our hormone of stress. And stress plays a very large role when it comes to memory. Whether you had stress as a child... stress when you're 30... stress when you're 60 – that all plays a role.

We can measure your stress hormone, cortisol. It is a salivary test, and if cortisol is not normal, the good news is we can normalize it and balance it in every single person.

CUT TO:

JACOB TEITELBAUM: Estrogen, testosterone – use the bioidentical forms of these hormones, and at optimized levels. Don't use the synthetics. They're poison.

And·also, when it comes to the reproductive hormones – just because the patient is not reproducing anymore doesn't mean your body doesn't need them. Optimize testosterone in men and women, and optimize using bioidentical estrogen and progesterone. You'll find a major difference in how you feel.

CUT TO:

PEGGY AND LEE IN THE STUDIO:

LEE: So hormones are really important.

PEGGY: Hormones are important. Every doctor trained in the new way to treat Alzheimer's knows to look at hormones as one of the factors that can cause cognitive loss. And I just want to underline what Dr. Teitelbaum said about bioidentical hormones. He's telling us to use natural hormones, the same ones that are in our bodies. If you do that, the results are remarkable. Here's Dr. Bredesen again with a look at a real-life case...

CUT TO:

DALE BREDESEN: I'll give you the example of another person, a 75-year-old woman, a very intelligent woman, a professional woman, who had major, major problems with her memory. And in fact, her significant other said, "Your memory is disastrous."

She would go out and try to play golf or she would try to do her job, and could not remember anything. She took online testing. She was at the 9th percentile. She'd always been very intelligent. She was at the 9th percentile for her age.

She went on this program. She's now at the 95th percentile for her age on her memory scores. She actually wrote to me and said that she was out playing golf with her friends, and she could say, "This person had this score, and this person had this score..."

PEGGY: Oh, beautiful.

BREDESEN: ..."and I had four shots here, two shots there..." you know, that sort of thing. So things started coming back. When she came to us, evaluation revealed that she had low vitamin D, low estradiol, low progesterone, low pregnenolone, low thyroid... all of these things. She had a very typical story for type II Alzheimer's disease, and she's actually done very well.

And interestingly, her significant other, when she started on this, said, "Okay, you've gone from disastrous memory to just plain lousy."

And then later (because he didn't really pull punches) he said, "Your memory's back to normal," which it is.

PEGGY: Another Alzheimer's survivor.

BREDESEN: She's done very well.

CUT TO:

PEGGY AND LEE IN THE STUDIO:

PEGGY: So infections, mold, environmental toxins, hormone levels, low levels of BDNF, blood sugar and diabetes... there are many things these cutting-edge doctors look at when they see an Alzheimer's patient.

LEE: I can see why a drug isn't likely to solve Alzheimer's disease or memory loss.

PEGGY: That's right. There are too many underlying causes. You have to look at the whole picture. The drug companies have been totally focused on getting rid of beta amyloid plaques. That's why the drugs have all failed. There are many different causes for brain plaques and there is no one drug that's going to address all these causes. Dr. Bredesen and I had a chat about this, let's take a look...

CUT TO:

PEGGY: As you're explaining the complexity of this, it just becomes so obvious why all these amyloid trials have failed. The amyloid is there for a purpose. The purpose is different in each of the cases, and it's brought on by underlying factors. Taking an Aricept is not going to optimize your vitamin D, or fix what's wrong with your thyroid, as an example.

DALE BREDESEN: We made a list of features for what a perfect drug for Alzheimer's would look like. What would it have to do? What are all the different mechanisms it would have to address? And there are about 100 different things on our list that it would have to do.

It has to normalize all your hormones, right? It has to optimize all your nutrition. It has to do all these things for you – increase your NGF, and your BDNF, and all these things. That's a very tall order for one drug.

So I happen to think drugs for Alzheimer's are a wonderful idea, but do it on the background of the overall program. If you're going to remove someone's amyloid, great. First remove the reason that they're making the amyloid. Because we've had people come through who've had some amyloid removed and done worse, because the amyloid is there as a protection. You have to first look at what's actually causing this to be made. Once you do that, you're in much better shape.

CUT TO:

DAVID PERLMUTTER: The brain doesn't decline just because one thing is askew. Multiple things conspire to create an environment in which the brain then is unable to thrive. That said, you have to target as many of those entities as possible, if you're going to reverse Alzheimer's disease.

CUT TO:

PAMELA WARTIAN SMITH: Our goal is to look at the cause of the problem, and not just treat symptoms, and to develop a very customized and personalized approach for every single patient.

PEGGY: Well, that's why you do personalized medicine. Now I get the title. So the fact that you want to get to the root cause is a little bit different, because many times we see doctors treating symptoms, and not going deeper into finding out what's causing these symptoms.

SMITH: That's really the good news in medicine now and in the coming years. We really can look at the cause of many disease processes, including cognitive decline.

PAMELA WARTIAN SMITH: Memory loss really is a multi-factorial problem, and so we just go down the road of looking at each of these in a very customized approach.

CUT TO:

NORMAN DOIDGE: Dr. Bredesen's shown that there are multiple paths to Alzheimer's, for instance. So it stands to reason that there would be different approaches to each of them. And what we know from his work, and what I find in my work, is that most people with a brain problem need multiple approaches. That's where the phases of neuro-plastic healing may be helpful, because it tells us, are we addressing these various things?

In Alzheimer's, we know there are many biochemical things going wrong. There are hormonal things. There are inflammatory problems, etc.

CUT TO:

PEGGY AND LEE IN THE STUDIO:

PEGGY: So, two big takeaways here: There's no one, simple "cause" of dementia. Alzheimer's disease or dementia can be caused by a number of different things, or combinations of different things. And no one drug is going to treat all of them.

LEE: And I'll add a third takeaway, if I may. Even if such a miracle drug could be developed, wouldn't you rather get to the root cause of what's making you sick?

PEGGY: Right, we don't want Band-Aid solutions. We want to regain our brain.

LEE: Catchy phrase! I noticed Dr. Doidge used a phrase people may not be familiar with – "neuro-plastic healing." What's that all about?

PEGGY: I'm so glad you asked. Getting the interview with Dr. Doidge was a terrific coup for me. He's the author of many articles and two best-selling books on breakthroughs in brain therapy. One of them is called *The Brain That Changes Itself: Stories of Personal Triumph from the Frontiers of Brain Science*.

LEE: Wow! I love it. Stories of personal triumph are just what we want. If I get sick, I want to be "a story of personal triumph."

PEGGY: Yes. Dr. Doidge is a worldwide expert on neuro-plasticity – the ways we can actually alter our brains with just pure energy – light, electrical stimulation, or brain exercises. Not by ingesting drugs, or surgery, or supplements or even changing the way we eat. Just with different forms of energy. But let's go to our next clip and let him explain...

CUT TO:

NORMAN DOIDGE: It's a property of the brain that allows it to change its structure, its physical structure, and its function in response to mental experience and activity.

So what you do, what you experience, what you think, even what you imagine can actually change your brain structure. And what we've been doing in the last while is using our understanding of plasticity to help people with various kinds of brain problems.

PEGGY: When you say it changes the structure, if we're going to look at imagery of a brain, it's going to look different after you've done these techniques that we're going to describe today. The brain is actually physically going to change.

NORMAN DOIDGE: Yes, yeah.

PEGGY: Okay, that's exciting stuff.

DOIDGE: We can now get inside the deepest part of the brain, for instance, through the tongue. By stimulating the tongue with certain electrical patterns, we can get into the brain stem. And the brain stem is a massive control center for the brain and the body, and we influence that.

We can get into the brain and influence it with light, and with sound, and even with movement, if we know what we're doing.

CUT TO:

LEE AND PEGGY IN THE STUDIO:

LEE: It sure is exciting stuff. Did Dr. Doidge give you any examples of neuro-plastic therapy?

PEGGY: Absolutely. The interview is packed with information. It airs on Day 9 of this series, and I hope everyone makes sure to tune in. One of the things Dr. Doidge talked about was the use of cold lasers – lasers that don't cut and burn the way hot lasers do. In early animal experiments, scientists showed that cold laser light could heal wounds or even cause hair to regrow.

Let's listen again to Dr. Doidge...

CUT TO:

NORMAN DOIDGE: They started shining light on things like E. coli – small organisms – and they found that light could do many, many things. They found that light could actually help the production of DNA. It could lower inflammation in bodies. It could eliminate pain.

So people started using light for the body. There's one case I described where one of the physicians was using it for someone who had suffered a neck injury in a car accident. The physician put light on the back of his neck. That man also had had a stroke which narrowed his field of vision.

And in the course of his treatment for his sore neck, his field of vision, which was like a keyhole, started to expand. And the physician realized, "My goodness, I'm also very, very close to the occipital cortex, the part of the brain that processes vision. Maybe light is actually helping vision."

And a number of clinicians started increasingly using light for things like migraine headaches, and ultimately for traumatic brain injuries.

What we believe is happening here is that there are certain specific frequencies that are in these lasers that promote healing and decrease inflammation. And they also influence the mitochondria, which are the powerhouses in the cell, so to speak. They produce the energy to re-energize.

CUT TO:

PEGGY AND LEE IN THE STUDIO:

PEGGY: This is very new and cutting edge. In one part of the interview, Dr. Doidge describes how you can get into the brain stem and affect it by stimulating the tongue with certain electrical patterns. The brain stem is a massive control center for the brain and body, and they can influence that through the tongue. He also talks about a type of auditory therapy, using music, that successfully treats children with autism.

LEE: I've heard of that. It's available from some doctors already, right?

PEGGY: Yes, it is. Researchers have figured out that autistic children just process sound differently from the rest of us. Sounds that don't bother us are extremely frightening and disturbing to them. But using a type of music therapy they can be trained to process sound the normal way.

CUT TO:

NORMAN DOIDGE: And as they start to develop the auditory zoom – and sometimes it can take several days – kids will do amazing things. They will turn to their father for the first time and hug him. And their speech will improve, and they will lose their sound sensitivities.

CUT TO:

LEE AND PEGGY IN THE STUDIO:

PEGGY: It's an exciting breakthrough. Another thing Dr. Doidge talks about is exercising the brain, brain-training programs.

LEE: Do those work? I've heard mixed reports. Some doctors tell patients to work crossword puzzles to keep their brains nimble. But it really doesn't do much good.

PEGGY: No it doesn't. When it comes to brain exercises, Dr. Doidge told me they tend to all get lumped together, and anything that has to do with the brain and some kind of computer is called a brain exercise. But there is a brain training program that DOES work and Dr. Doidge told me about it in the interview. Let's have one more sneak preview...

CUT TO:

NORMAN DOIDGE: The brain needs to maintain itself, just like the heart. You know, to maintain your heart, you want to do some interval training, or you really want to work up a sweat and challenge it from time to time. Walking is fantastic, but to really get into top shape, you've got to do some exertion.

And the same goes for the brain. You can't spend a lifetime replaying skills you've already mastered, or you can't spend 30 years of middle age replaying mastered skills, and expect to maintain your brain function.

What has been shown persuasively is that people who are, let's say, 70 who have age-related cognitive decline and who do these brain exercises can start to function the way they did when there were 60 or younger, maybe even 55, maybe even younger, in some cases, and that it generalizes.

CUT TO:

PEGGY AND LEE IN THE STUDIO:

LEE: I'd love to take ten years off the age of my brain. What does he mean when he says "it generalizes"?

PEGGY: He means that the effects carry over into everyday life – and they last. For example, after the training, studies have shown elderly people have fewer car accidents. The whole interview airs on Day 9. Don't miss it. And that last clip reminds me of something similar Dr. Amen said about learning and changing. Let's roll it...

CUT TO:

DANIEL AMEN: When you stop learning, your brain starts dying. You need to be engaged. Now, at some point I may retire.

PEGGY: I can't picture that.

DANIEL AMEN: But I want to retire and do something else. I'm going to do something interesting, something that keeps me passionate and engaged – and I am now, with what I do, so I can't imagine not doing that. But that's really critical, new learning. And not doing things you already know how to do.

For example, I know how to write and I know how to teach, so I need to be doing different things that stretch my brain in new and different ways.

CUT TO:

PEGGY AND LEE IN THE STUDIO:

LEE: We've got to challenge ourselves. We've got to keep growing.

PEGGY: We need to challenge ourselves and learn new things. It literally reshapes our brains. You can see it in brain scans. As Bob Dylan said, "He not busy being born is busy dying."

LEE: The next 11 days are a great chance to get busy being born. They're packed with life-changing information. Tell us more…

PEGGY: I've barely scratched the surface of what these eleven interviews contain. For example, a lot of people worry about genetics. Maybe some of our viewers have heard of the APOE4 gene, which increases your risk of Alzheimer's. Several of our doctors go into that in detail and you'll have a good handle on genetic risk after you watch this series. The good news is, bad genes aren't a death sentence. Here's what Dr. Amen had to say…

CUT TO:

DANIEL AMEN: Genetics. If you have Alzheimer's or a form of dementia in your family, you have a higher risk. Now, it's not a death sentence. It's a wake-up call. I have heart disease in my family. I have obesity in my family. I don't have heart disease myself, and I don't have obesity. Why? Because I don't engage in the behaviors that are likely to trigger my genetic risk.

CUT TO:

PEGGY AND LEE IN THE STUDIO:

LEE: Yes, if we've learned one thing today, it's that so much is under our control.

PEGGY: You can change your brain, but you have to have a plan. And one of the most important parts of the plan is getting a good night's sleep. It turns out that if we don't sleep enough, or if our sleep is poor quality, it brings on dementia. Our risk of dementia goes way up.

The brain repairs itself at night. That's when a lot of housekeeping goes on – dead cells and waste matter are cleaned out. It's also when our brain moves our short-term memories to the parts of the brain where long-term memories are stored. If we don't sleep well, those memories are lost, and we can't remember what we did yesterday.

LEE: So our brains are doing a lot of work at night. They're busy.

PEGGY: Yes, they're busy. Our brains are just as active when we're dreaming – during the REM stage of sleep – as they are when we're awake. And REM sleep is just one of four stages of sleep you have to go through for the brain to do all its housekeeping. If you don't sleep straight through for two or three hours at a time, without waking up, then the brain's work doesn't get done. And you have to go through the complete four-stage cycle several times a night to maintain optimum brain health. Sleep affects our bodies in ways you wouldn't imagine. But let's let the doctors tell us...

CUT TO:

DANIEL AMEN: When you sleep, your brain cleans and washes itself. So if you don't get seven hours at night, the cleanup crew doesn't have enough time to clean up the mess that you made during the day.

CUT TO:

PAMELA WARTIAN SMITH: Sleep is key for memory. When you don't have good sleep hygiene, meaning that you don't sleep at least six and a half hours to eight hours a night of good, restorative sleep, it drives up your blood sugar. And it's one of the mechanisms that causes memory loss.

CUT TO:

DAVID PERLMUTTER: The other thing that's really vitally important, as it relates to brain health, is getting restorative sleep. It's so highly underrated, the notion that sleep makes you feel good – great. But sleep is a brain tonic, and it's really important to recognize that the quality of our sleep matters in ways that are almost indescribable.

People may think they're sleeping well, but in reality, the five hours that they're getting a night is not enough. Or they may think they're sleeping for eight hours, but in reality, that sleep is very interruptive, and not restorative.

CUT TO:

LEE AND PEGGY IN THE STUDIO:

LEE: Okay, I see what they mean. So tell us what we can do to sleep better. What are we going to learn from these interviews that will help us sleep?

PEGGY: Well, I invited our old friend Dr. Michael Breus for a return engagement. He's a sleep expert who's written two books and has appeared on Dr. Oz more than 30 times. Dr. Breus was a big hit in our first interview series.

In this new interview he comes loaded again with tips on how to rejuvenate your brain with better sleep – with a special focus on circadian rhythms, which turn out to be hugely important. For example, he tells us the first two things we should do when we wake up in the morning. It's surprising, but the key to a good night's sleep is often what we do at seven in the morning! Here's just a taste...

CUT TO:

MICHAEL BREUS: If you remember, everybody's got an internal biological clock called their "circadian rhythm." And it turns out there's three or four different circadian rhythms out there.

Once you know what that circadian rhythm is, you can actually figure out the exact right time of day to do whatever it is you want to do, whether it's read a book... get new information... have a cup of coffee... go for a run... have some mental clarity... be creative... sell... buy. Whatever it is you want to do, there are actually specific times in your biological rhythm when you're better at it, and I've figured out a way to identify them.

CUT TO:

PEGGY AND LEE IN THE STUDIO:

LEE: So if you follow Dr. Breus's lead and get in tune with your circadian rhythms during the day, you'll be all ready for a good night's sleep.

PEGGY: That's right. And there's much more in this interview, which airs on Day 4. He outlines a routine to follow the last hour before bedtime that will help you sleep – including a very clever trick to switch off your worries for the night. It's a way to put your cares behind you for just those eight hours or so you need to sleep. This is a super interview. Let's look at his advice on just one thing, sleeping pills...

CUT TO:

PEGGY: Let's talk about sleeping pills.

MICHAEL BREUS: Right. There are lots of medications out there, and if you read the labels, almost all of them either make you tired or make you unable to sleep, right?

PEGGY: Not good.

MICHAEL BREUS: Not good in either direction, so I'm a big "less medicine is better" kind of person. I'm not saying don't take medicine. I'm not saying be afraid of medicine. Medicine can be extremely helpful, but just speak with your doctor about getting the lowest effective dose.

Sleeping pills are a whole different ballgame. There's a lot, a lot, a lot of people out there who are taking sleeping pills, and there are all kinds.

PEGGY: We're talking about prescription sleeping pills.

MICHAEL BREUS: We are. Well, we can talk about either. We can talk about prescription sleeping pills, or we can talk about over-the-counter sleeping aids.

PEGGY: Let's begin with the prescription ones, because millions of people are on them.

MICHAEL BREUS: They are. Other than thyroid medication, it's actually one of the most heavily prescribed classes of medication out there.

It turns out there are three different classes of sleep medication. There's what are called the "non-benzodiazepine hypnotics" – Ambien, Lunesta, those types of medications.

PEGGY: Okay.

MICHAEL BREUS: There are the benzodiazepines, which were originally anxiety medications, like Valium, or Xanax, or Restoril. There's another class of sleeping pills which are actually anti-depressants – Trazodone is a big one. Celexa is one that can actually be quite helpful for sleep.

The question becomes, do you really need a sleeping pill?

I'm of the belief that some people out there may have a "broken sleeper," right, that switch in their head that makes them fall asleep. But most people don't have "a broken sleeper." Very few people have that where it's broken.

CUT TO:

LEE AND PEGGY IN THE STUDIO:

PEGGY: You can see he's really thorough. If you watch this interview on Day 4 and put the tips to work, you'll sleep better. And if you sleep better, your risk of dementia and a whole raft of other medical problems will go down. And if you're already experiencing memory loss, you'll get better. It's a must-see interview.

LEE: I know a lot of people neglect sleep. We're up late on the computer or smartphone or watching television. And some people are up often during the night because of pain or the need to go to the bathroom. A lot of people have sleep apnea, and don't know it

PEGGY: Lack of sleep is an epidemic. Dr. Breus – and other doctors in the series, too – talk about the problems you just mentioned and others. This is a problem you may be able to solve, and regain your brain, quite possibly without spending a dime.

LEE: How I wish we'd known all this when my mother had Alzheimer's 19 years ago. What a difference it would have made. My brother and sister and I had to watch her sink out of sight, like a ship going down beneath the waves.

Sometimes she wouldn't know who we were. Other times she kind of knew I was someone she should know, but she couldn't quite remember who I was. She couldn't remember my name, same way I might meet someone on the street that I haven't seen in a couple of years, and not remember their name.

The worst thing is she was frightened all the time. I could see it in her eyes. There was this terrible fear because she didn't know people, she didn't know what was happening to her. Her identity got erased, but her body was still around. They kept the dementia ward locked so people couldn't get out. That's because these patients literally don't know who they are, and they wander off and get lost.

And this isn't unique, it happens to millions of people. There are more than five million people with Alzheimer's in the United States. You can multiply my mother by millions. And most doctors STILL tell the families it's hopeless, there's nothing you can do. And that's not true anymore. Even advanced cases can recover some function, and many people come all the way back. They regain their brains. And the sooner you get started, the better.

Do you have any idea what it's like for people when their mother knows them again, knows their name, after months or years of being lost in fog? That happens now, it's happening all the time.

That's why I produced this series and why it's so important to get people to watch it, as many people as possible.

PEGGY: The title of this series says it all: Regain Your Brain. You can do that. The knowledge is here, the technology is here. The answers are here. You just have to use them.

I absolutely believe – I know – the next eleven days can change your life and the lives of people you love for the better. Please don't miss even one day. Every episode is packed with life-saving answers, including new scientific breakthroughs that are turning this whole field upside down.

Tomorrow we kick off with the first interview, Dr. Dale Bredesen, the man who was the first to publish the results of a human trial in which Alzheimer's disease was reversed. He explains how he did that, and how his protocol can work for you. By the way, he has already trained hundreds of doctors in the protocol and he's adding more all the time, so these are solutions you can get now, almost anywhere. This interview sets the table beautifully for the whole series. Don't miss it.

LEE: Wonderful! We have to leave it there, Peggy. Thank you so much for being here.

PEGGY: Thanks, Lee, it was my pleasure.

Interview with Dale Bredesen, M.D.

PEGGY SARLIN: Hello, I'm Peggy Sarlin, and today I'm in San Francisco, where I have the great honor of speaking with Dr. Dale Bredesen, the first person to publish a study documenting how he reversed Alzheimer's – dramatically so, in many cases.

His new book, *The End of Alzheimer's* – Did you get that? *The End of Alzheimer's* – describes in detail how he did it, and how you can do it, too.

Dr. Bredesen is the Founding President of the Buck Institute for Research on Aging, and he's a leading expert on the mechanics of neurodegenerative diseases. You are going to be so encouraged by this interview, and I think you're going to find extremely valuable Dr. Bredesen's insight that Alzheimer's is not just one monolithic disease. Instead, it's three distinct, separate syndromes, and that matters a lot in terms of how you treat it.

So this is really valuable information. Welcome, Dr. Bredesen.

DR DALE BREDESEN: Thanks very much, Peggy.

PEGGY: So in 2014, you published your groundbreaking study that showed how you reversed Alzheimer's in nine out of ten people. That's a small sample, admittedly. But you've been busy since then, so tell us, what are you doing now? What's the scope of what you're up to?

DR BREDESEN: Right. There are several hundred people now on the protocol, and it is a personalized protocol based on each person's genetics, biochemistry, infectious illnesses exposure... a whole series of things. We've published a follow-up paper, and we're now working, actually, on a third one that is expanded in terms of the number of overall people.

But we have seen unprecedented improvements in many people with pre-Alzheimer's, so-called "MCI" or "SCI," as well as those with Alzheimer's disease. And we're learning lessons, such as, some of the people that we thought were too late for the program have actually done quite well on the program.

So we're learning specific things about how to optimize the program.

PEGGY: I love the phrase you used. I remember when we first spoke, you used it: "unprecedented results." That's really the key. What you're doing, your protocol, is yielding unprecedented results. That's where the future is.

DR BREDESEN: That's right. In general, we were all taught that Alzheimer's couldn't be prevented; the cognitive decline associated with Alzheimer's could not be reversed. But that's no longer what we're seeing.

And this is really part of a bigger picture. This is part of a revolution in medicine, where we are moving from 20th Century medicine to 21st Century medicine. In 20th Century medicine, which was what we doctors were all taught, and which is what's being practiced in most places, the emphasis is on "what." What is the diagnosis? Is it heart failure? Is it Alzheimer's? Is it cancer?

In 21st Century medicine, it's completely different. The emphasis is on "why." Why did you get this illness? And as you might imagine for complex chronic illnesses like Alzheimer's, cancer, cardiovascular disease – and those are now the three leading causes of death in the United States – the causes are turning out to be complicated. So there are many, many different things that contribute to cognitive decline.

PEGGY: I think that's such a central insight in your book, talking about the complexity of it – that Alzheimer's is not one thing. You divide it into primarily three things.

DR BREDESEN: Right.

PEGGY: And maybe you can help us understand that. I want to say, what really struck me is that in your description of each of these three types, they manifest so differently.

DR BREDESEN: Right.

PEGGY: They manifest at different ages, different decades of life, and the cognitive problems that they create are also distinctly different. They're different animals. So help us understand that.

DR BREDESEN: That's exactly right. What we found was actually diametrically opposed to the claim that when your brain makes amyloid, this is a bad thing for your brain, and this causes your brain to get damaged, and we want to get rid of that bad stuff.

What we found is, in fact, the opposite. Amyloid is a protective response that, in fact, we make in response to three different classes of pathogens and insults. And certainly, other groups, such as Dr. Moir and Dr. Tanzi from Harvard, have shown that there is an antimicrobial effect to amyloid, which fits into this whole, overall picture perfectly.

What happens is that we get exposed to a number of things during our lives, and as part of a protective response, we make the very stuff that the pathologist looks at and says, "Oh, you have Alzheimer's disease." This is a protective response to three different things.

Number one, which gives you type I Alzheimer's, is inflammatory, so – inflammation. It can result from foods that you ate – trans fats, too much sugar – things like that actually cause inflammation; or you can cause inflammation by having chronic pathogens – herpes simplex virus type I is one of them, for example. Lyme disease, borrelia, other tick-borne illnesses, specific fungi and molds, specific bacteria, P. gingivalis, which comes from your mouth...

So perhaps we shouldn't be surprised. Things in this area especially, or that are systemic can find their way into your brain. And guess what? Part of the protective response to these is what we call Alzheimer's disease.

So getting rid of this amyloid response is a little bit like sending the police home when there is crime. Yes, if the police are there all the time, if you're living in a police state, there are going to be good people who, unfortunately, may get hurt. But they're there for a reason. So before you send them home, you want to find out why they're there to begin with, you want to find out what is causing this. So that's what we call type I Alzheimer's.

Type II Alzheimer's is very different, as you said. This is what happens when you have a withdrawal of trophic supporting influences on your brain, and there are lots of them: Vitamin D, estradiol, testosterone, nerve growth factor, brain-derived neurotrophic factor, Vitamin B 12, other nutrients...

All these are critical for providing the very support your brain needs to keep up the synapses. So literally, your brain is looking at the situation in terms of, "Here's what we'd like to have. We'd like to have this network. Here's the network we can actually afford, based on the nutritional or hormonal or other support we have."

So now, as you start taking things away, it's no different than what happens in a company: If you don't have the right things coming in, you're going to have to downsize. And what's the first thing that your boss tells you? "We can't hire any new people."

So that's what your brain says. "We're going to keep the stuff we have. We're still going to know how to drive. We're still going to know how to play tennis, or what have you. But we can't bring on new memories."

And when that happens, it's the canary in the coal mine, telling you, "Okay, you're at the limit. You need to look at why it is that you can't add new memories." And that's what we call type II, or atrophic. Type I is the inflammatory; type II is the atrophic.

Now, if you have a sugar-related problem, which is where you get prediabetes, and you get insulin resistance, that's actually type I.5, because the sugar-related problem gives you both inflammation, and it gives you the trophic withdrawal, because your body doesn't respond normally anymore to insulin. So that's what we call type I.5.

Then type III is a very different illness. It looks different. It acts different, and you must treat it different to get the optimal outcome.

That is toxic Alzheimer's disease. This is where you are exposed to specific toxins, and – guess what? – your brain makes the amyloid also to bind to these toxins, be they chemical toxins like mercury or copper, or be they biotoxins like mycotoxins, that is,mold-related toxins.

Surprisingly, it turns out that mold species, especially things like Stachybotrys, and Penicillium, and Aspergillus, and Chaetomium... these all make toxins, neurotoxins that damage your brain. Your brain responds by making the protection, amyloid.

And doctors typically look at the brain and say, "Oh, this person had Alzheimer's disease, you know. We don't know why they had it." Well, no, now we do know why they had it. We can now look at these different parameters and determine why the people actually got this problem.

So that's type III Alzheimer's, and it looks very different because type I and II typically start with memory loss, so-called "amnestic presentation." The symptom is that people have trouble learning new things. Type III is different, because it typically starts with executive dysfunction: trouble with planning, trouble with calculation, trouble with visual perception, trouble with word findings, so-called cortical symptoms, so it's a different type, and is often found in younger people. We see a lot of people who are in their early 50s who are getting this.

When I trained in medicine, we didn't see anybody in their early 50s with Alzheimer's disease. Now this is coming out of the woodwork. We're seeing this all the time. We estimate, just based on the percentage of people who have this, compared to the other two types, there are probably at least 500,000 Americans who have type III Alzheimer's disease. It's turning out to be surprisingly common.

And of course, as you might imagine, many people will have some contribution from type I, maybe a little from type II, and then some from type III as well.

PEGGY: Right.

DR BREDESEN: Many people have mixed causes, and you need to address all the contributors to make these people better.

PEGGY: I think what you just told us highlights how complex this is, but the approach has been, "We're going to find the magic pharmaceutical pill."

DR BREDESEN: Right.

PEGGY: And there've been something like 300 trials of drugs. They've all failed, and considering what you just laid out, it almost seems, well, of course they'd fail. Look how complex this is. Look how many inputs there are to making this happen.

So, let's take a little time... I think people will want to know more – let's go over each one again and help people understand. Alzheimer's I...this is your own term for it? If you'd go to your doctor and say, "I've got Alzheimer's I," would they know what the heck you're talking about?

DR BREDESEN: Alzheimer's I, or type I Alzheimer's – no, most doctors would not know what we're talking about.

PEGGY: Did you dub it this?

DR BREDESEN: Yes.

PEGGY: Okay.

DR BREDESEN: I wrote the paper and published it on looking at the different subtypes.

PEGGY: Okay, so type I Alzheimer's, in Dr. Bredesen's terminology...

DR BREDESEN: Right.

PEGGY: ...is brought on by inflammation.

DR BREDESEN: Yes.

PEGGY: And the inflammation could be caused by – what? You mentioned a couple of different things. One of them is a poor diet.

DR BREDESEN: Yes.

PEGGY: What's the amyloid plaque trying to respond to... If you eat lousy, lousy food – junk, junk, junk, junk food...

DR BREDESEN: Yes.

PEGGY: What's the amyloid attempting to do? Does it cool down inflammation? How is amyloid a response to junk food?

DR BREDESEN: I'll explain. It's a response in that it is being told there is an ongoing inflammatory state. So imagine that you have a signal that says, "Okay, war is coming." Then you're going to get the troops ready. You're going to do all the things that get you ready for the coming onslaught. Similarly, the amyloid is there because it's expecting that there are going to be pathogens.

PEGGY: Oh, it's expecting pathogens.

DR BREDESEN: Inflammation is associated with microbes, and a common example is found if you look at people who have leaky gut – and I'm sure you've heard about leaky gut. It's turning out to be more and more common. It's turning out to be a bigger and bigger problem, and a common cause related to things like arthritis, cardiovascular disease.

And in this case, it's the same sort of story: chronic inflammation related to cognitive decline. In leaky gut syndrome, you breach your gut, and you now are filling your blood with pathogens, with fragments of pathogens, things like lipopolysaccharide, pieces of bacteria and things like that. So your body is now in a state of fire, a state of inflammation, trying to deal with that. And your brain is doing the same.

One of the ways we look at amyloid now is a little bit like an electrified fence. Imagine that you have barriers that are set up to be immovable. Your blood-brain barrier, your gut-blood barrier are specific barriers at specific locations.

But now what happens when those barriers are breached? Now you have to have a mobile barrier that says, "Okay, we're going to pull back the troops. We're going to pull back into the fort. We're going to downsize, but we're going to put up this electrified fence, and if they try to come across, they're going to be killed."

So to some extent, we're looking at Alzheimer's more and more as a mobile barrier to microbes and other things coming from inflammation.

PEGGY: When you were describing that, it was like a war game.

DR BREDESEN: Yeah.

PEGGY: Your body's doing this war gaming, and the amyloid is this weapon, this strategic weapon your brain can deploy.

DR BREDESEN: That's exactly right.

PEGGY: So okay, let's say you've had a lifetime of poor eating. Your brain's inflamed. It's on fire.

Your brain says, "Oh, there's more bad foods coming. There's probably a leaky gut. It's going to send me all these yucky microbes, and I'd better make some amyloid here."

What age is that going to start manifesting? What decade, typically?

DR BREDESEN: Well, interestingly, it's been shown that everybody over the age of 40, if their brain is stained for amyloid, has some amyloid plaques – everybody. So to some extent this is like looking at cholesterol. You know, some people have more and some people have less, but it's not something that you don't have.

It's just a question of how much, and it's a question of, do you continue the inflammation, and do you continue this in a way that you're now doing downsizing, downsizing, downsizing...? Or does it plateau? So basically, everybody over 40 has some amyloid in their brains.

PEGGY: But in terms of actually manifesting, to the point where somebody comes in and says, "Ooh, Mom's acting really weird" – what age would that be, typically? When it's a case where the inflammation has been incited by poor food choices?

DR BREDESEN: Right. It's a very good point. There's a huge difference between people. Some people will start to have problems with inflammation in their 60s and 70s. The typical person we see who's beginning to have symptoms is in their 60s for type I; is in their 70s for type II; and is in their 50s for type III. That's just a general rule.

PEGGY: That's general, but...

DR BREDESEN: But we see people outside that. But certainly, the bell-shaped curves for each group are different. We tend to see it earlier in the type IIIs, then the type Is. And then the type IIs are the latest ones, typically.

PEGGY: So if somebody comes in who's type I... maybe we should ask here: How do you know it's type I?

DR BREDESEN: We know that it's type I by using a computer-based algorithm we've created that looks at 150 different parameters and then tells you what percentage is type I, I.5, II, III. You can tell, basically, that it's type I – if it is type I – based on inflammatory profile.

For example, people who have multiple monoclonal – multiple autoantibodies. If you have people who have high hs CRP, that is, high-sensitivity C-reactive protein. That is something that goes up...

PEGGY: An inflammatory marker.

DR BREDESEN: ...right, when you have an inflammatory marker. Interleukin 6 is another one that's common. Tumor necrosis factor alpha – these are all things that come on with systemic inflammation.

PEGGY: Now give us a sense of what you do to help these people. Tell us a story, somebody who came to you...

DR BREDESEN: Right.

PEGGY: What were they showing that you determined was type I, and how did you get them better?

DR BREDESEN: Okay, we had one person who came in a few years ago who had classic difficulty with what he called "senior moments" (and this is discussed in the book a bit), and who had difficulty with his job, functioning in his job, difficulty with remembering appointments. And both parents had passed away from Alzheimer's disease.

He turned out to have the most important indicator of genetic predisposition, which is APOE4. He then had a well-documented Alzheimer's, with PET scan, both amyloid PET scan, and so-called "FDG PET scan," documenting that he was in the early stages of Alzheimer's.

He had an hs-CRP – which should be less than 1.0 – his was 10. So he had ten times as much as the upper limits of what you should have. He went on our program and after about three months, clearly improved.

He's now about three years out and doing very, very well. And when he's gone off the program, he's done less well, and when he's gone back on, he's done well again. And his numbers have come back.

So as the metabolism goes, so goes the cognition. Part of the issue here is to identify what's causing this inflammation. In his case, he had a horrible diet.

PEGGY: Horrible diet.

DR BREDESEN: Horrible lifestyle, and was literally giving himself Alzheimer's disease.

PEGGY: Well, your book has a scary chapter called "How To Give Yourself Alzheimer's" that basically describes, you know, most people's lifestyle.

DR BREDESEN: Right.

PEGGY: You made an important point there. You said, "When he's on the program, he does well, and his cognition comes back. When he goes off the program..." So we need to let people know this is not a magic pill. It's a program, and what does the program look like?

DR BREDESEN: Right. This is not a silver bullet. This is silver buckshot. So it is targeted. And of course, part of 21st Century medicine is precision – or targeted – medicine. If you're looking at a cancer, you look at the specific things that are causing the cancer, the entire genome, and you address the ones that are changed, that are actually giving you the illness.

This is no different. We identify the different things, and you want to find out what's actually causing this ongoing inflammation. Is this specific pathogen-associated? If so, you need to deal with those pathogens. Is this a breakdown in your immune system dealing with these? If so, you need to enhance immune function. Is this due to a genetic change? People with specific genetics tend to have difficulty handling certain pathogens, so you want to identify that.

And then, of course, are there specific things in the diet that are actually causing this ongoing inflammation? As you know, processed food, GMO-related foods, the so-called "SAD – standard American diet" – is a pro-Alzheimer's diet.

So here's part of the chapter: if you want to give yourself Alzheimer's disease, then one of the many things that you want to do to give it to yourself is to follow the standard American diet.

PEGGY: Oh, that's scary. No, we don't want to give ourselves Alzheimer's. We most certainly don't.

DR BREDESEN: But that also is the good news. You can prevent it by staying away from that, and you can prevent it by following your biochemistry. As we tell people, everybody knows that when you get to 50, you have a colonoscopy. And everybody over 45 should have a "cognoscopy."

And it's relatively straightforward: you want to know your blood testing for your genetics and your biochemistry. You want to know where you stand. You want to know if you have chronic infections, and you want to know where you stand genetically, and then also, where you stand with your performance.

Doing that, the reality is, Alzheimer's should be a rare disease. It's a very common disease now. It should be a rare disease – and it can be, with what we know today.

PEGGY: Well, you make the point that everybody knows somebody who survived cancer, but we haven't known anyone who survived Alzheimer's.

DR BREDESEN: Right.

PEGGY: And now we do, thanks to your work. So, the person you just told us about who's now come back to full cognitive function as a result of following your program...

I just want to say personally, in your book, you have a moving section about somebody whom you treated who wrote to you what it feels like to come back from dementia, a detailed description.

DR BREDESEN: Right.

PEGGY: And she used the term "awakening." And I found that somewhat beautiful, because my book is called *Awakening from Alzheimer's*, and the video series is called *Awakening from Alzheimer's...",* and that's been my premise from talking to doctors such as yourself: that it's possible to awaken from this. And that was the term she used, so I like that.

DR BREDESEN: Absolutely, absolutely. And that's the thing, that's the reason everyone should be coming in earlier and earlier – and preferably, be on prevention, but if you've missed the prevention part, and you've started to have some symptoms, then come in and get on the program earlier. Get yourself evaluated so that you can turn this around quickly.

And as you said, she did a beautiful job with this. Now, her father was in very, very late stages, so she had seen this before. When she started having problems, she wasn't sure if this was the same thing, but she started realizing after a while she was going through the same sorts of things he had.

PEGGY: Right.

DR BREDESEN: She was having many of the same sorts of symptoms. And she actually went to a major university on the East Coast and was evaluated, and she was shown to have some abnormalities already there when she was still relatively young.

So then she ended up going on the program over the next several months. And it typically takes three to six months. She did very, very well. She was able to see what it would feel like to be heading down toward dementia, and then what it felt like when you come back out of that.

PEGGY: An awakening.

DR BREDESEN: As you've said, it was an awakening. She could really see what she felt like. She could remember things like the mistakes she made. She described, for example, going through the toll booth and saying the wrong thing, instead of saying "carpool." And so each thing where she would make mistakes... have trouble with her memory... have trouble with reading... difficulty with languages that she had known... difficulty with interacting with her children, with helping them... all these sorts of things were starting to disappear.

And then, seeing what it felt like when she now was able to do all these things again. And then going back to the University, being evaluated again, and having them show that, "Yes, now you are testing back into the normal range."

PEGGY: Well, that's why I said right at the outset that I think people watching this are going to be so encouraged, exactly because of stories like this. You're bringing Alzheimer's survivors into the world.

Now let's move on to type II, but first we'll recap type I for people, just so they remember. It's brought on by inflammation, and the amyloid, which is really quite strategic. I'm getting this respect for amyloid now from your work. It knows how to strategically position itself. The amyloid in inflammatory Alzheimer's is there to cool things down, and take on the nasty microbes that are coming your way.

DR BREDESEN: It is part of your immune system, and specifically, your immune system has two parts: the innate part, and the adaptive part; innate being the old part, the part that is more generalized, and the adaptive is the more specific part. So this is the more generalized part of your immune system, and it's responding to problems.

PEGGY: Okay, so that's type I, and we have a sense of it. Now, type II Alzheimer's... what is it?

DR BREDESEN: Type II is very different. It results from not being able to support the network structure that you have in your brain.

You have to remember, you've got nearly one quadrillion synapses in your brain, about 10^{15} synapses, so it takes a lot to support all this. And if you start decreasing trophic support – whether it's hormonal, whether it's nerve growth factor, or brain-derived neurotrophic factor or others, or whether it's nutritional – when you're deficient in any of these things, you can no longer support that sort of network. And in fact, you then start a strategic downsizing.

In fact, somebody asked me, "Why would a strategic downsizing lose memories for you? Because isn't that something important?" Well, yes, but in fact, what you have before is even more important. For your whole life, you have collected only the most important things: how to do your job, how to speak, how to calculate, how to write, how to read... all these things.

So if I asked you, "Would you rather forget those things, or would you rather forget the "Friends" rerun from last night?" Of course, it's easy, right? Because each new thing that you're learning is less likely, overall, to be as important as all the things you've learned before.

So the first thing that goes is the ability to acquire new information. That's when you want to jump on things and make it...

PEGGY: The short-term memory that we associate with Alzheimer's.

DR BREDESEN: Exactly. Consolidation of new memory. Exactly right. So in order to keep your other memories you sacrifice the ability to assimilate new ones...

Interestingly, when I wrote the paper on these different subtypes that you can see, you can recognize them. When you have larger biochemical data sets, you can see these different subtypes, because you can read the molecular tea leaves and see who's got type I, who's got type II.

Well, guess what? It turns out the Ayurvedic physicians were a couple thousand years ahead of me. They had already described dementia that is associated with so-called "hot" or "pitta" characteristics in a person, and "vata," which is dry. So vata, their vata type of person is basically what we call type II, or atrophic. These are people who don't have the trophic support for the neuronal network.

PEGGY: Just a little vocabulary question here... Most of us laypeople aren't familiar with the term "trophic" or "atrophic." Can you define it, since that's what you're calling it, it's important that we understand what that word means.

DR BREDESEN: Yeah, this is a really good point. Trophic is essentially life-supporting, so it involves giving – whether it's to a neuron, or another type of cell – giving support to allow the functioning and the survival (and often, the differentiation as well) of a specific cell.

So we look at this whole brain, the whole network, as having support. And when we talk about trophic support, there are dozens and dozens of things that are involved with that. For example, your nerve growth factor is actually made through a number of multiple cells in your body.

Your brain-derived neurotrophic factor – same story. And there are dozens of these trophic factors.

Then there are also things that have a trophic effect, such as estrogen, testosterone, pregnenolone, in some sense, neurosteroids, DHEA and things like that.

PEGGY: Hormones.

DR BREDESEN: Hormones. Free T3, a thyroid hormone, is very important. All of these trophic factors provide support, trophic support, providing for life-giving support of the cells and the connections in the brain.

And then there are nutrients also. Vitamin D is a good example. Problems occur if you drop your vitamin D too low. It's associated with cognitive decline, epidemiologically. So all of these things provide this trophic support to the brain.

PEGGY: I guess the question I have, then, is why do you have low trophic support? It seems, if you say it's nutrition for the brain, that seems to go back to type I, which you get if you didn't eat good food. Or is the source of the problem not the diet? Why is this different?

DR BREDESEN: It's a very interesting point you bring up, and that's why we have what we call "type I.5," which has some of type I, and some of type II. A good example: people who've consumed too much simple carbohydrate, too much sugar, so they now have chronically-high insulin levels.

They develop what's called "insulin resistance." But they also have the inflammation from the sugar itself, and from the modified proteins that occur because of these high concentrations of sugars. So you have both an inflammatory component, and a trophic component. You're no longer responding as well to your insulin.

So you're absolutely right. A poor diet can lead to type I, because of the inflammation, but it can also lead to type II because of the decrease in trophic support. That's a good point.

PEGGY: What else might lead to type II?

DR BREDESEN: For example, people who have thyroiditis, who drop their thyroid levels... people who go through menopause, especially when they experience a rapid decline in trophic support. That is very important. People who have hypovitaminosis D, that is, people who aren't getting enough vitamin D. And as you know, this is very, very common throughout the world.

These things all can contribute to this type II. You don't see much inflammation in type II. And in fact, often people will actually have lower inflammatory status than normal. But nevertheless, there is a decrease in cognition, and a decrease in the overall synaptic network – but again, by a different mechanism in type II than in type I.

PEGGY: So when you were talking, I got a picture. You said, "the decreased hormones in midlife, and low vitamin D." A woman may be going through hormonal change in midlife, and not going outside to get some sun, and next thing you know, Alzheimer's type II. Is that a reasonable scenario?

DR BREDESEN: Exactly. Exactly. And in fact, it's been shown by nice studies out of the Mayo Clinic that women who had early hysterectomies with oophorectomy, with loss of the ovaries, and who did not receive hormone replacement therapy, in fact doubled their likelihood of developing Alzheimer's later in life.

PEGGY: Ooh, and they don't know that.

DR BREDESEN: And of course, most of the people who've had the hysterectomies and oophorectomies are not aware of this.

PEGGY: No.

DR BREDESEN: So this is, again, the type II Alzheimer's disease.

PEGGY: This is the type II. When does this manifest? What decade? And what are the telltale kinds of cognitive signs that you see?

DR BREDESEN: Right. The type II tends to be an amnestic presentation.

PEGGY: What does that mean?

DR BREDESEN: People have trouble with storing new memories. They typically will present to the doctor in their 70s, but they've often had some trouble from even their 60s, and sometimes even their late 50s.

What we call "brain fog" associated with menopause often goes away. But in fact, as PET scan studies have shown, for example, many of the same sorts of changes in the same sorts of areas of the brain can occur during menopause, and can occur later during Alzheimer's disease.

So the stage may be set by this sudden, relatively rapid drop in hormonal support for the synaptic structure in the brain, with full-blown Alzheimer's disease later on. So typically, we see these people come to the doctors in the 70s.

The way they look is often very strikingly just lost. This is the most pure example in terms of a memory loss. People will be able to drive their cars, get around. They don't get lost. They can calculate. They can do their checkbooks. They can do everything, and so no surprise, often their spouses will say, "Well, you know, you're having trouble." And they'll say, "Well, I can do this, this, this..."

It's like, they can still do all these things, and they'll say, "Well, you know, you're not perfect either." Which is, of course, often true.

PEGGY: Sounds like every marriage.

DR BREDESEN: Exactly. So these people often do very, very well, and one thing that happens is memory loss. That's the first thing.

Now, the problem, of course, is that you're now undergoing a downsizing. If you don't do something about it, you do start having other problems. But initially, it is pretty much a pure memory loss.

PEGGY: And here, we return to the role of amyloid as this strategic genius.

DR BREDESEN: Yes.

PEGGY: So the amyloid's being expressed to say, "I'm not getting enough nutrition, not enough fuel. I'm going to have to start rationing things. Okay, I'm going to shut down this function... I'm going to try to gunk over this section here, which contains what you had for breakfast this morning." And eventually will go, "I'm gonna shut down, you know, your daughter's name, or what a key is for, if it keeps on this way..." But it's rationing energy...

DR BREDESEN: Right, slowly.

PEGGY: ...saving it for more important needs... Is it rationing energy to tell your heart to keep pumping, and you to keep breathing, those kinds of...?

DR BREDESEN: No, no.

PEGGY: No, it's not for that.

DR BREDESEN: No, it's not – as far as we know, it doesn't have any effect on the heart. It is changing your overall neural network. But what happens is, the amyloid that you mentioned is a little piece of a bigger protein, and this is called "amyloid precursor protein" or APP.

APP turns out to be a little bit like the CFO in your company, the chief financial officer. It's looking at many different inputs. You know, what came in through this account? What came in through here? Did we do our online marketing? Did we sell stock? Did we have bonds? All these things.

In a similar way, APP is looking at whether there was enough estradiol. Was there enough testosterone? Was there enough vitamin D? Was there enough NGF (neural growth factor), BDNF?

It is an integrating receptor that literally acts like a switch. When there is enough to support it, it is cleaved at one site, and produces two pieces of protein, two peptides, that actually tell you to upsize, and to go ahead and make and keep these interactions, the synapses.

On the other hand, the same protein, this same APP, when it's cleaved at three sites, produces four pieces that all are saying something. These are like memos, they're like memos going out from the CFO. There are two of them that are for the public, and two of them for their internal consumption, giving directions to the cell.

And what they're saying is, "We can't afford what we're doing. We are now in the red, so we're going to have to downsize," as you said earlier.

And it's actually quite functional, because you still keep all the things you've learned throughout your life at the beginning, but you simply can't learn new things, as that brain function shuts down. APP starts to do the downsizing.

You have quite a nice program which tells you, "Get on it now. You should now be treating things so that your functional loss doesn't progress, and hopefully, you get back the memory that you've lost."

PEGGY: Tell us a good story about somebody who came to you with type II from not enough of the trophic factors.

DR BREDESEN: Sure, yes. Right. I'll give you the example of another person, a 75-year-old woman, a very intelligent woman, a professional woman, who had major, major problems with her memory. And in fact, her significant other said, "Your memory is disastrous."

She would go out and try to play golf or she would try to do her job, and could not remember anything. She took online testing. She was at the 9th percentile. She'd always been very intelligent. She was at the 9th percentile for her age.

She went on this program. She's now at the 95th percentile for her age on her memory scores. She actually wrote to me and said that she was out playing golf with her friends, and she could say, "This person had this score, and this person had this score..."

PEGGY: Oh, beautiful.

DR BREDESEN: ..."and I had four shots here, two shots there..." you know, that sort of thing. So things started coming back. When she came to us, evaluation revealed that she had low Vitamin D, low estradiol, low progesterone, low pregnenolone, low thyroid... all of these things. She had a very typical story for type II Alzheimer's disease, and she's actually done very well.

And interestingly, her significant other, when she started on this, said, "Okay, you've gone from disastrous memory to just plain lousy."

And then later (because he didn't really pull punches) he said, "Your memory's back to normal," which it is.

PEGGY: Another Alzheimer's survivor.

DR BREDESEN: She's done very well.

PEGGY: And it's somebody who experienced awakening from Alzheimer's.

DR BREDESEN: Exactly.

PEGGY: We haven't talked too much about what the program is, but you can kind of get a sense from what you're saying. In type II, you're going to optimize vitamin D. You're going to balance hormones.

DR BREDESEN: Right. What you do is, we look at all of the things that are involved with the downsizing side, which is what we call "synaptoclastic." When people look at osteoporosis, for example, they look at two kinds of cells – osteoblastic and osteoclastic – so, osteoblasts and osteoclasts. The blasts are the ones that are making the bone, and the clasts are the ones that are reorganizing. They're basically pulling back.

We see the exact same thing with Alzheimer's. There's a set of signals that are making and storing memories. These are synaptoblastic, literally, and include all the things we've been talking about. And then, there's another set that are pulling back.

And it's normal. You know, we think we should never forget anything. Not true, you should forget things. We all forget actively, you know, the seventh song that played on the radio on the way to work yesterday.

So there are active things that we should be forgetting. We're keeping the most important things in our minds so that we can do things like remember what words to say, and talk to friends, and do our jobs, and read, and write, and all those sorts of things. This is from the beautiful balance of synaptoblastic and synaptoclastic. So there is a balance there.

What we do with all these people, whether it's looking at risk and trying to prevent or reverse cognitive decline, is to decrease the synaptoclastic signals and increase the synaptoblastic signals, because everybody with Alzheimer's or Alzheimer's risk is on the wrong side of that balance.

If you have too much synaptoclastic activity and not enough synaptoblastic activity – it's the same idea as osteoporosis. We're now going to do everything possible with all the signals, all the right things that you need to do to give yourself the synaptoblastic activity and reduce the synaptoclastic activity.

PEGGY: As you're explaining the complexity of this, it just becomes so obvious why all these amyloid trials have failed. The amyloid is there for a purpose. The purpose is different in each of the cases, and it's brought on by underlying factors. Taking an Aricept is not going to optimize your vitamin D, or fix what's wrong with your thyroid, as an example.

DR BREDESEN: Right. Right.

PEGGY: Okay, that's type II. Type III – very different.

DR BREDESEN: Right.

PEGGY: Tell us about type III.

DR BREDESEN: Just to finish up the last sentence you said – sorry – we made a list of features for what a perfect drug for Alzheimer's would look like. What would it have to do? What are all the different mechanisms it would have to address? And there are about 100 different things on our list that it would have to do.

It has to normalize all your hormones, right? It has to optimize all your nutrition. It has to do all these things for you – increase your NGF, and your BDNF, and all these things. That's a very tall order for one drug.

So I happen to think drugs for Alzheimer's are a wonderful idea, but do it on the background of the overall program. If you're going to remove someone's amyloid, great. First remove the reason that they're making the amyloid. Because we've had people come through who've had some amyloid removed and done worse, because the amyloid is there as a protection. You have to first look at what's actually causing this to be made. Once you do that, you're in much better shape.

I think that bringing the programs we've developed together with specific drugs will be a very powerful tool. Again, personalized, programmatic, looking at a precision approach to what's actually caused the problem.

So you asked about type III – very different disease. And in fact, what we're finding is that type III is a closer relative to what's called "Lewy body dementia," and there are about a million Americans who have Lewy body dementia.

PEGGY: Oh, yes.

DR BREDESEN: It's the second most common cause. Type I, type II, and type I.5 are over here. They're more typically amnestic in their presentation. Type III is more like Lewy body disease.

And actually, it typically presents non-amnestically. Now, some of these people do end up with memory problems as well. That happens. These are people who typically start young, often in their late 40s to early-to-mid 50s. They have problems with organizing. I hear people who will not be able to pack their bags anymore and get out the door. They can't follow directions anymore. They can't figure out how to put things together.

They are much more impaired than the type II people who can do everything well but just can't remember what they had for breakfast. But they can do everything else well. They can drive. They can get themselves around. They can do their jobs – all that stuff.

The type IIIs are much more impaired, and they typically have a more general abnormality when you look at their scans. They have less of a brain downsizing and more of random damage, in keeping with the fact that all of the people with type III turn out to have toxic exposures, be they biotoxins, or chemical toxins, or physical toxins – EMFs and things like that.

In fact, people who have type III usually turn out to have biotoxin exposure, and sometimes things like mercury, or high copper-zinc ratios and things like this.

These people start with difficulty with either organizing or word-finding problems, so-called "primary progressive aphasia," visual perception problems, praxis problems, specific learned programs, dyscalculia, that is, problems calculating, one of the most common things.

People will say, "Gee, I just, I couldn't, I couldn't figure a tip anymore," and that's often the first thing that goes. These are so-called "cortical abnormalities," as opposed to the more hippocampal abnormalities seen with the memory.

Often these people have some depression with their problem as well, whereas the other ones less commonly have depression as a presenting characteristic. Often, with these people who are type III, especially because they're young, the doctors will say to them, "Well, you're too young to have Alzheimer's. You're just depressed. We'll give you an antidepressant." And then it'll take a few years before anyone realizes, "Now wait a minute. These people really have Alzheimer's disease."

When you do the appropriate scans, they really do have Alzheimer's. They have amyloid in the brain. Their PET scans are abnormal. Their amyloid PET scans are abnormal. Their FDG PET scans are abnormal. Their cerebrospinal fluid is abnormal. Very compatible with Alzheimer's disease, but it is a type III Alzheimer's disease.

The amyloid seems to be there to bind to these various toxins and to interact with them, and again to protect the brain from things like mercury and mycotoxins.

So with these people you need to look at what toxins they've been exposed to. What is present? Why did you make this amyloid binder to these toxins?

PEGGY: So what are some of the common toxins that people are exposed to that incite this?

DR BREDESEN: The most common ones turn out to come from biological sources, from organisms. So – mycotoxins, things like Stachybotrys, a strain of mold; and Penicillium; and Aspergillus; and Chaetomium. All of these things and others will produce neurotoxins such as okra toxin A, and Trichothecenes, Aflatoxin, Gliotoxin... These are all biological toxins produced by molds.

PEGGY: By molds.

DR BREDESEN: By molds. And then there are some where Lyme inflammation-associated infection seems to be common. And interestingly, you'd think, "Well, Lyme, shouldn't that give you type I?"

PEGGY: Yeah, that was my next question.

DR BREDESEN: These people have some of that, but often there's not a lot of inflammation there. This is a chronic infection that's been going on for years, and there's not a lot of inflammation, so there's not a lot of the type I. There's really more of the type III.

So, yes, Lyme disease, mycotoxins... And then chemical toxins, things like mercury, whether you get inorganic mercury from your fillings or organic mercury from eating seafood. Either one of those can give you something that is, for all the world, Alzheimer's disease, positive scans, typically diagnosed as Alzheimer's disease. And yet, when you deal with the mercury, these people get better.

And then there are other toxins, and actually, Dr. Joe Pizzorno is doing some very interesting work looking at other toxins associated with Alzheimer's disease, and with cognitive decline, and finding additional organic toxins, things like DDE, and DDT, and even things that have been brought up in the past, things like aluminum. People have kind of gone away from the idea that aluminum has anything to do with it.

PEGGY: Yes.

DR BREDESEN: But his new studies are suggesting that maybe aluminum has been a contributor in some people. We're still learning what are all of the different toxins that can lead to cognitive decline.

PEGGY: So in type III, the damage tends to be more random. I mean, type I and II, it shows up in the hippocampus, the traditional area associated with Alzheimer's. In type III, which is caused by a toxin, it's scattered throughout the brain? It's a random distribution, almost, or what...?

DR BREDESEN: It doesn't seem to be completely random, because when you do the PET scans to look at the actual metabolism, you still do see temporal and parietal.

It's seen in temporal and parietal abnormalities. But their symptoms are typically more of a biparietal. They have things that are parietal lobe abnormalities. On the scans they often do show some atrophy throughout the brain, but the initial abnormalities often seem to be biparietal.

PEGGY: You mentioned executive function. "I can't pack my suitcase. I can't organize. I can't..." It was a different manifestation than type I and type II. It can show up earlier, because you can be exposed to mold at any time in your life. If you're living in a moldy house, I mean, theoretically, a kid could have it.

DR BREDESEN: Absolutely.

PEGGY: I mean, if a kid's living in a moldy house the symptoms could occur. What's the youngest person you've ever seen with this?

DR BREDESEN: Well, people can get it in their 20s and 30s. In general, when you're young, you have other manifestations of exposure to the same molds.

So, for example, you will have a family where the child might get asthma, one parent might get cognitive decline, and the other parent might get fibromyalgia, that sort of thing, and that can all be from mold exposure. So they have different ways that their different bodies are dealing with the same problem.

PEGGY: That brings us to something I don't think we've talked about, which is the genetic predisposition to Alzheimer's, because here we're talking about how people individually react to something like the exposure to mold. That's not type IV Alzheimer's, with a genetic origin? Where does having the marker, the APOE4 marker – where does that place you in this, in this realm of the three types?

DR BREDESEN: Right, right. There are hundreds of genes associated with risk for Alzheimer's. The most common is APOE, as you alluded to. And if you look at our population, as a nation we have about 325 million Americans. A quarter of them, about 75 million, are APOE4-positive, meaning they have a single copy of APOE4, and that puts them at increased risk.

If you have zero copies of this gene, your risk is about 9% for your whole lifespan. If you have a single copy of APOE4, it's about 30%, and if you have two copies – and there are seven million Americans who have two copies of APOE4 – then your risk is over 50%. So if you have two copies it's more likely that you will get it than that you will not get it during your lifetime.

And this is why we suggest that everybody find out your status and get on prevention early. This should be a rare disease.

PEGGY: But what type are you going to get? Let's say you have the two copies, which raise you to 50% risk, I think you said. What's going to happen to you?

DR BREDESEN: Right, right. The people who have APOE4 typically get type I, or 1.5, or II, and not III. And interestingly, the people who get type III are often APOE4-negative.

So when you have someone who's APOE4-negative who gets it at a young age, who starts with problems with calculation or organizing, and has no family history, that's typically type III Alzheimer's disease, especially if they have some depression. All these things go together.

So what happens with APOE4? We discovered that if you look at APOE4, one of the interesting things it does is it actually reprograms your cells, and makes them more pro-inflammatory. Well, that's great for our forebears, who came down out of the trees between five and seven million years ago. They needed this pro-inflammation to deal with eating meat that was uncooked, with microbes in it, stepping on dung, walking across the savanna...

PEGGY: Doesn't sound very appetizing.

DR BREDESEN: No, that's right – but with all the things we went through all those years ago, it helped to have this pro-inflammatory state.

Now, of course, as we get older, it turns out it's not so helpful. But it can be a good thing when you're young, especially if you're living in a squalid environment.

PEGGY: Right.

DR BREDESEN: But it's not such a good thing when you're older. They have a pro-inflammatory state, and that's why they can present with type I. Again, people who eat sugar and things like that are also more at risk for type I.5, and they also have some risk with the atrophic response, so they can also have a greater likelihood of type II, but not so much with type III. Not to say they cannot get it, but you're actually more at risk to become a typical type III if you are APOE4-negative.

PEGGY: That's interesting. Who would have predicted that, right?

DR BREDESEN: Yeah.

PEGGY: So maybe we should talk a little bit now about cases. Tell us a story of somebody who came to you with type III. And I know that's not an easy type to treat, the exposure to toxins.

DR BREDESEN: Exactly. Type III has been the toughest one, because you have to identify all the exposures. And the surprise is, people end up having a combination or a multiple of these.

There's a suggestion... we don't understand this yet, but there's a suggestion that once you essentially have lowered your ability to fight one of these, that others actually come on more easily. We don't know this yet, but it's looking more and more suggestive that in fact, we're keeping all these things at bay, and once you have one, you may be more susceptible to another.

Here's a woman, for example, who went to a national center for Alzheimer's disease when she was in her mid-50s, and she was having trouble with organizing things, trouble with calculating, trouble with doing her job.

And she was found to have early Alzheimer's disease. She ended up having an MRI scan that actually showed her hippocampal volume at less than one percentile, so it was very, very shrunken there. But she was having trouble with things beyond just memory.

She ended up being diagnosed with multiple mycotoxins. She ended up having mold exposure. She ended up having chronic and undiagnosed Lyme disease, chronic and undiagnosed babesios, which is a parasite that's also given to you by ticks.

PEGGY: Oh, my gosh.

DR BREDESEN: And she turned out to have some problems also with glycotoxicity as well, and turned out to be APOE4 single copy.

So she was living in a home. Her husband actually is a physician, and he took her to another home. You can get what's called "ERMI score," which is related to the Environmental Protection Agency, the EPA. It's EPA-related mold index – or Relative Mold Index, ERMI.

As Dr. Shoemaker, who's done a tremendous amount of work on mold-related illness, has shown, if you have the propensity for having illness with respect to mold, then you need to live in a place or home where the ERMI score is less than two.

Hers was 6 1/2, which is far too high. Her husband moved her to a new home without checking the ERMI score. He figured because it was a newer home, everything would be okay. It turned out that her ERMI score at the new home was seven, so it was worse than the other home.

PEGGY: It was worse than the original home.

DR BREDESEN: And while they were doing this, he started having his own symptoms. Now, his turned out to be more pulmonary symptoms. He was treated. He's done better, and she went to see Dr. Ross, who's superb at dealing with these sorts of problems.

She went on a program, first involving identification of the various things she'd been exposed to, and then followed by a program that dealt with each of these, including enhancing her immune system... including removing the exposure... including specific atrophic support.

So once you're now removing the exposure, you want to have the ability to clear those toxins, and one of the useful things is to increase your glutathione level, which was done for her.

When her glutathione level would go up, in fact, she would do better for a period of time, until it would start to go down again, and then she would do not as well. And then it would be increased again, and she would do well again. So repeatedly, as her glutathione level would increase, she would do better.

Her husband also noted that as she would exercise, she would actually do better. As her bioidentical hormones were improved and optimized, she did better. She made gains, and the gains were very clearly associated with improvement in her MoCA, her Montreal Cognitive Assessment, and in her ability to interact with other people.

One of the really common things people say, as people start getting better, is that their socialization ability improves. You can see they're sharper. They're more on the ball. They can interact better with you. They can follow directions.

We had another woman who came in who was having all sorts of problems, and improved her scores as well. She was having trouble with spatial orientation, and after she was on the program for several months, she got in the car and her husband said, "Oh, unfortunately, I forgot the directions." She said, "Oh, don't worry. You take a left here..."

It was 15 miles to get to where they were going. "Take a left here, right here, left here, left here, right here..." And he looked at her and he said, "You haven't been able to do that in years."

Other people will say they got interested in reading again, because before they were treated they weren't able to follow things and to understand what was going on. And they will get interested in reading, and talking about their reading once again.

PEGGY: Again, you're bringing us the survivors of Alzheimer's, hers from a type III. So I guess we've gone through the three types, and we've given people kind of an overview. What should they do? If somebody's watching this and they are concerned about themselves or somebody else, what's the next step? Do they contact you? You can't treat the whole world.

Talk to the families who are watching about what they should be doing with this information.

DR BREDESEN: Right. There are three things you can do. Number one, start by looking at my book, because this breaks down why you need to have these various tests. That gives you some background.

Second thing, you look at the websites, www.MPIcognition.com or www.drbredesen.com , and they go through these various things as well.

And then, the third thing, talk to a practitioner who is aware of this program. We've now trained 450 practitioners in seven different countries and all over the United States. There will be over 1,000 trained by the end of this year, so they can talk to you about the program and about my...

PEGGY: So how do I find that doctor?

DR BREDESEN: You can do that, actually, on the website. There'll actually be a map so you can see who's close to you.

PEGGY: And that website is MPIcognition.com...

DR BREDESEN: Or drbredesen.com.

PEGGY: Or drbredesen.com. And I can find locally, hopefully, a doctor who's been trained in your protocol, the Recode Protocol.

DR BREDESEN: Right, right.

PEGGY: I've also heard – because we have an Awakening from Alzheimer's Facebook page, a private group, and we've been talking about this – that some people have gone to doctors that you've trained, and they've also had consultations via Skype.

DR BREDESEN: Yes, a number of people will do this. You can have a consultation over Skype to learn more about what are the steps to take...

Understandably, this is part of a major and fundamental change in our medical system that's happening, the difference between 20th Century medicine and 21st Century medicine. So understandably, people are skeptical at the beginning, and saying, "You know, is this really important?"

I got one letter from a couple in Canada, and they had taken the paper, a paper that I wrote, to their doctor, and he said, "I'm too busy to read anything, so I don't want to see this." And they started – well, they started, "Could we talk to you about some of this?" And he said, "I don't hear anything about nutrition, because doctors don't do nutrition."

Well, if you're a doctor and you're not doing nutrition, then you're not in the 21st Century, because it is an important part of what's happening in the entire system.

These are complex chronic illnesses that we're dealing with, unlike pneumococcal pneumonia of 100 years ago. These are very different situations, whether you're talking about cardiovascular disease, or cancer, or neurodegenerative disease, or other common illnesses.

PEGGY: That's why you use the term "programmatics."

DR BREDESEN: Right.

PEGGY: Did you make that term up?

DR BREDESEN: I did, yes.

PEGGY: Programmatics means creating programs for people to follow.

DR BREDESEN: Right, yes.

PEGGY: It's not the pill, it's the program.

DR BREDESEN: Yes, and pills are fine, but do it with the program.

PEGGY: Do it with the program.

DR BREDESEN: ...so you can get the best benefit. Again, this is part of precision medicine. It's

21st Century medicine, to understand all of the contributors. When we have a very complicated physiology, don't think that you're going to get it just by looking at someone's sodium and potassium. You need to look at a much larger data set.

And Silicon Valley will be very, very helpful at looking at these larger data sets. They're already looking at things like the whole genome. That's actually a relatively simple thing, compared to all the different physiology and metabolism and lipidome, and all these sorts of things that are critical for how we are dealing with disease, and our long-term health.

PEGGY: So let's just wrap up here by saying to the families watching, they go to your website. They go to drbredesen.com, MPIcognition.com.

DR BREDESEN: Or a practitioner, yeah.

PEGGY: They find a practitioner. Then just give us an idea – what's going to happen? What's he going to do?

DR BREDESEN: He or she will meet with these people and look at all the different things that are either contributing to risk for cognitive decline, or to actual cognitive decline... will look at a larger data set, and then be able to tell you, through our computer-based algorithm, "What are my risk factors?" Or "What are the things that are actually driving the decline?"

Which is what you need to know.

And then from there, a personalized program will be generated. Each person is different.

PEGGY: Each person is...

DR BREDESEN: What's good for this person here is not necessarily what's good for this person here. You need to address what's causing your risk, or your decline.

PEGGY: Hence the personalized medicine, 21st Century medicine. Okay.

DR BREDESEN: Exactly.

PEGGY: So we're getting ready to wrap up here, but if you could just leave us with a little pep talk, maybe, for everybody, everybody who's got a brain, about the importance of the care and tending of it, of the cognoscopy, and of just being aware at a young age of what we should be doing.

DR BREDESEN: Right. As you know, your brain is important. And if that's not working, then it doesn't really matter if everything else is working, because if your brain's not working, you're in trouble. So it's an important thing to take care of, and unfortunately, you can have problems with it that have been going on for years that you were unaware of.

So we recommend that everybody, especially people who have a family history of Alzheimer's disease or dementia, and especially people who have any suggestion that there is some decline...

And by the way, if you've recently said, "You know, I really want to get on prevention because I'm concerned." It often turns out on evaluation that they were already beginning their cognitive decline. And it can be hard to recognize at first. Alzheimer's can be, unfortunately, a seductive killer. It's not something that's obvious, sometimes, at first, until it's further along.

So we recommend that everybody over 45 have a cognoscopy, and that really means looking at your function. You can do this. There are online tools that are very inexpensive. In fact, you can do MoCA score for free, and do it in 15 minutes, and just see where you stand.

Then you can get some blood tests, and again, the physicians who are trained in this can give you specific blood tests that will tell you, "Where do you stand with your type I, with your type I.5, with your type II, with your type III. Where do you stand with your systemic inflammation? Where do you stand with your glycotoxicity?"

For example, what's your fasting insulin? Everybody should know their fasting insulin. It's an important contributor to cognitive decline. If yours is drifting up, it's good to know that early on, before it's done damage to you.

What's your status with respect to your trophic support? What is your estradiol hormone level? What is your testosterone? What is your Free T3, Free T4, reverse T-3...? All these things can tell you, can help to tell you whether you are at risk.

And then type III – do you have the specific genetics that are characteristic of being sensitive to those toxins, and do you have exposure to those toxins? That can be picked up fairly easily.

So all of these things are critical to know, so that you can make sure where you stand. And as I said earlier, Alzheimer's disease should be a rare disease if all of us do the right things.

PEGGY: Well, you are helping to make it so, and we certainly thank you, and wish you enormous luck with your work, and with training a new generation of doctors to help us prevent this.

DR BREDESEN: Thanks.

PEGGY: Thank you so much for watching. I hope you learned today from Dr. Bredesen, who's really one of the major figures of our time in leading this fight against Alzheimer's disease. And I hope you find the information useful for you and your family to reverse cognitive damage, and to prevent it from happening in the first place. Thanks for watching.

Interview with Daniel Amen, M.D.

PEGGY SARLIN: Hello, I'm Peggy Sarlin, and today I'm in Costa Mesa, California, at the Amen Clinic with Dr. Daniel Amen. And you know Dr. Amen from his ten best-selling books, and from his public television series.

He's a board-certified psychiatrist – double-board certified – who's been called "the most popular psychiatrist in America," and he's the Founder of the Amen Clinics. There are now seven of them across the country. And – of crucial importance to what we're going to talk about today – the Amen Clinics have built the world's largest database of functional brain scans, more than 135,000 of them.

Now, Dr. Amen has written a really great new book called *Memory Rescue*. There's so much actionable information in it that I just want to dive right in so you can start learning. So, welcome, Dr. Amen.

DR DANIEL AMEN: Thank you, Peggy.

PEGGY: You know, in your book, you write that 75% of older Americans report memory problems, and once you reach age 85, you have a 50% chance of dementia. So those are some pretty scary numbers there.

But you've come up with what you call an "insanely simple idea" to counteract this problem. So tell us your insanely simple idea.

DR AMEN: If you want to keep your memory healthy, or even get it back if you think it's in trouble, you have to prevent or treat all of the risk factors that steal your mind. So, I mean – super simple – we know what steals your mind, and almost all of the risk factors are preventable or treatable, even the genetic risk factors. We're finding that the things I talk about in *Memory Rescue* are even more helpful for the people who are most vulnerable.

So how exciting is that? The fact that you are not stuck with the brain you have. I think our big databases taught us that you can make your brain better, even if you've been bad to it, and I can prove it. You know, when it comes to the imaging, we have done thousands of after-scans after we saw troubled brains.

Just last week, a really well-known best-selling author came to see us two years ago, and her brain was just a mess, and she was a mess – problems with memory, and focus, and irritability, and not being able to get work done. And she's 46.

By doing all the things we asked her to do, when we did her two-year follow-up scan, we found she is dramatically better, and her brain is dramatically better. And she has Alzheimer's disease in her family. At her first scan, our reaction was, "Oh, you're headed to the dark place." Because we can tell...

PEGGY: You can see it.

DR AMEN: ...decades before you have any symptoms. And the exciting thing is, she's not stuck with that brain. She's not stuck with that trajectory. You just have to be serious, and you have to have a plan.

PEGGY: You have to have a plan. Your book gives us the plan, but we should say right off at the beginning that if you want to save your brain, you are going to have to do this plan. You're actually going to have to do things. There isn't going to be some magic pill. You are going to have to be motivated.

So maybe one of the things to help people get motivated at the start is, let's tell them some of the good things that will happen. We know they're going to get their memory back, but you mentioned also that she was less irritable, she had better focus, I bet she looked better... I mean, tell us some of the other good things that we can expect – to motivate us to do this plan.

DR AMEN: Well, you're thinner, you're smarter, you're happier, you're energy's back.

PEGGY: I love it already.

DR AMEN: Now, all of those are things that we really want. And again, it's not hard. I've been working with a group at Stanford on how people change their behavior. And you change it through a series of small decisions or tiny habits. And as we studied it, we went, "What's the most important tiny habit that you can have?"

And it comes down to asking yourself every day one really simple question: Is what I'm going to do today good for my brain, or bad for it? And if you can answer that question... Now, it requires knowledge...

PEGGY: You're giving us the knowledge.

DR AMEN: ...because a lot of people think that alcohol is good for their brain. The imaging work I do says no.

PEGGY: No, no.

DR AMEN: Forget it. It's not a health food. Some people think smoking pot is good for your brain.

PEGGY: That's one of my questions.

DR AMEN: The imaging work says, stop lying to yourself. It's bad for you.

PEGGY: Okay, good, I'm glad.

DR AMEN: Anything that makes you eat and causes you to be dumb is not a good thing for your brain.

But it's using that one little question that I've actually played at this game with my daughter since she was two. We call it "Chloe's game." She's 13 now. And the question is, "Is this good for your brain, or bad for it?" And she can answer the question in almost any situation she's in.

If I say, "Avocado," she'll say, "Two thumbs up. God's butter." If I say, "Blueberry," she'll put her hands on her hips and go, "Well, are they organic?" Because nonorganic blueberries have more pesticides than almost any fruit. And I'm like, "Of course, they're organic." She says, "Well, God's candy." I say, "Talking back to your redheaded mother." She'll say, "Way too much stress. Bad for you." Right?

PEGGY: So you said, "Every day, we're going to ask ourselves, 'Is this good for my brain?'" But actually we're going to ask ourselves that throughout the day, every time we face a food choice... every time we face, maybe, an interaction that might promote stress.

It's a constant question which we're probably not used to asking ourselves. We're not used to thinking, "Is this good for my brain?" Most of us are not programmed to think that way.

DR AMEN: Well, because nobody loves their brain. I mean, it's crazy.

PEGGY: You love your brain.

DR AMEN: I love mine, but very few people love their brain. And you know why – the reason is you can't see it. You can see the wrinkles in your skin, or the fat around your belly, and you can do something when you're unhappy with it. But because nobody looks at the brain, people don't fall in love with it.

And that's how I came to all of this, because I'm a psychiatrist, you know. Why do I care about Lyme, and mold, and making sure you're not overweight? That wasn't part of my training.

PEGGY: Right.

DR AMEN: But when I started doing imaging, I saw my brain at 37, and it wasn't healthy. And my 60-year-old mother had a better-looking brain than I did. I come from a very competitive family, and that just irritated me. I'm like, "Well, what can I do to have a better brain?" Well, you do the right things, and you don't do the wrong things.

Science has told us, "These things are really great for your brain, and these things aren't." Because with a better brain, everything in your life is better. Your relationships are better. Your health is better. Your money's better... because you make better decisions.

PEGGY: Decisions. I'm with you.

DR AMEN: Making decisions is a brain function.

PEGGY: It's a brain function. I love what you're doing, because you're helping us fall in love with our brains. You're giving us an appreciation for our brains so we love them, you know. That's good.

One thing you wrote in the book I found absolutely fascinating was that people are coming to you later in the game of cognitive decline because of GPS. I think that's important, so tell us about that. People need to hear this.

DR AMEN: I know. What a crazy thing. Thirty years ago, I would be in my office, and a wife would bring in a husband because he started crying. He couldn't find his way home in the city he'd lived in for 30 years.

PEGGY: Right.

DR AMEN: But now, because of our smart phones, you can just type in "home," and it will find your way home. So people are actually being diagnosed later than ever before, because of the assistance of technology. We can hide our problems more effectively.

PEGGY: That's – I think that's a crucial point. I don't think most people are aware of it, and obviously, we see the benefits of this technology. But the fact that it's disguising weaknesses we need to address is not well known, so I did want to start with that point.

So you've put together a program, The BRIGHT MINDS Program, and we should say it's a mnemonic device. Did I pronounce that correctly?

DR AMEN: Right, which is Greek for a memory.

PEGGY: It's a memory.

DR AMEN: A mnemonic device is how we help people remember things. You know, when you go to medical school, the first year you have to learn 50,000 new words, and new terms... arrgh!

PEGGY: It's hard to just hear you say that.

DR AMEN: So we came up with all sorts of memory devices, mnemonics, and so on... as I was thinking of the big risk factors that you need to attack to keep your mind healthy, or even rescue it, if it's in trouble.

There are 11 of them. And we've created a mnemonics program, BRIGHT MINDS, to help you remember them.

PEGGY: Let's go through them so people get a sense of the full scope of what this program entails, so they can get a sense of what they're going to do.

DR AMEN: But before we do that...

PEGGY: Okay.

DR AMEN: ...can I just talk about seahorses for little bit.

PEGGY: I know where you're going with this.

DR AMEN: It's really important to understand a part of the brain called the "hippocampus." It's on the inside of your temporal lobes. It's about the size of your thumbs, and the hippocampus is critical for memory learning and your mood. Hippocampus is Greek for "seahorse." In *Memory Rescue,* I talk a lot about the seahorses in your head.

PEGGY: Right.

DR AMEN: And actually toward the end of the book there's a story of Scarlett and Sam, the seahorse twins. It's really about what grows them and keeps them big, healthy and strong, and what shrinks them and makes them old, weak and frail.

The hippocampus is a very special part of your brain, because it's one of the few parts of your brain that continually makes new nerve cells, or new brain cells. There are stem cells in the hippocampus. A healthy hippocampus makes up to 700 new brain cells every day.

I think of them as 700 baby seahorses, and the question is, are you doing things in your life that encourage them to survive and thrive, or are you doing things that kill them off?

If you love yourself, you want to love your seahorses. And just remember that visual, if you will. Am I really taking care of part of me that is so special? It really holds the treasure chest of my most precious moments, and I'm not dumping it out because I just make bad decisions.

PEGGY: Well, the hippocampus is where Alzheimer's starts. It's absolutely...

DR AMEN: It's the first area of the brain that dies.

PEGGY: I've read a lot about this, but I learned something new from your book. Actually, this will bring us to the first letter in your mnemonic: "B" for blood pressure, right?

DR AMEN: Blood flow.

PEGGY: Blood flow. That's what I meant to say. So I learned from your book that when the blood-brain barrier starts to erode, starts to deteriorate, the first place that it starts to deteriorate is around the hippocampus. And that seemed to me to perhaps correlate with Alzheimer's, if that area is becoming more porous, more vulnerable.

DR AMEN: More vulnerable to toxins, more vulnerable to infections, more vulnerable to inflammation... And the hippocampus is just so special. I mean, all of your brain is important, but when it comes to memory, this is the area we know is critical.

PEGGY: So let's start with "B" – blood flow. What do you want to tell us about blood flow?

DR AMEN: "B" is for blood flow. Low blood flow is the number one brain imaging predictor of Alzheimer's disease.

PEGGY: That's what you're seeing on your...

DR AMEN: That's what we see on our brain scans. The scans we do here at Amen Clinics are called "SPECT," which stands for "Single Photon (piece of light)... Single Photon Emission Computed Tomography." It's basically a nuclear medicine study that looks at blood flow and activity patterns in the brain. And we can tell decades before you have any symptoms whether or not you're headed for trouble.

What are the things that make us vulnerable to blood flow problems? Blood pressure. Any vascular or heart condition will do it. Being sedentary.

PEGGY: Being sedentary.

DR AMEN: Caffeine constricts blood flow to the brain in a powerful way. Nicotine constricts blood flow to the brain. Having erectile dysfunction, because if you have blood flow problems anywhere, it means you're having them everywhere.

In *Memory Rescue,* we go through each of these risk factors and we ask, "Okay, which ones do you have? And how do you attack it?"

Obviously, you've got to get your blood pressure treated. If you have any vascular or heart condition, you need to be serious about treating them. So many people are not serious...

PEGGY: Right.

DR AMEN: ...about treating them, because they don't know their "why." They don't know why they want to be healthy. And exercise is probably the most powerful thing you can do to keep Scarlett and Sam, in your hippocampi, healthy

PEGGY: Your friendly seahorses.

DR AMEN: And it's not just any kind of exercise. It's coordination exercises, because they actually boost your cerebellum, in the back bottom part of your brain, which helps turn on your frontal lobe, so your judgment and decision making will be better. I like dance and table tennis, my favorite.

PEGGY: I noticed a table in the other room.

DR AMEN: Burst training is actually better than riding a bike.

PEGGY: What was that one? I missed that one.

DR AMEN: Burst training...

PEGGY: Burst.

DR AMEN: Or it's called "high intensity training."

PEGGY: That one I'm familiar with.

DR AMEN: Rather than just be on a bike for half an hour, it's much better to sprint for 30 to 60 seconds, and then go at a normal pace, and then sprint again for 30 to 60 seconds, and do that four or five times. Your metabolism will go up, but it's also been shown to increase blood flow, and to do better.

And then strength training – very important, even if you're a girl, even if you're 80. Don't hurt yourself, but the stronger you are as you age, the less likely you are to fall. We'll talk about that under "head trauma," but it also increases blood flow. So coordination exercises, strength training, high intensity or burst training.

It doesn't have to be hard. I'm a total believer in, "What's the easiest way I can get this done?"

PEGGY: Yeah, I love that.

DR AMEN: So I lift weights for about 35 minutes, twice a week. And I work out each muscle group, and at 63 I'm stronger than I've ever been.

PEGGY: That's good.

DR AMEN: But I'm not going to be in the gym for an hour. I also walk a lot, because I listen to books on tape, and I like it. But while I walk, I burst. So I'll walk, and then I'll walk as fast as I can, and then I'll go back to normal... And I play table tennis, and I do it because I love it, and I know it's good for me.

PEGGY: So we know that if we want to really address blood flow issues, we're going to do these exercises, and we're going to think of it as making baby seahorses in our hippocampus.

DR AMEN: Right.

PEGGY: We're giving birth to new brain cells, and that's why I'm going to get off the couch, and do what I don't want to do.

DR AMEN: Because you don't want them dying.

PEGGY: No, you do not want them...

DR AMEN: You don't want the babies dying.

PEGGY: No. No.

DR AMEN: This is all about love.

PEGGY: Love. Love your brain.

DR AMEN: And people don't get it. The attitude is, "Oh, I don't want to do this. Oh, I don't want to do that." And I'm thinking, "Stop being a four-year-old." I'm thinking, "Come on..."

This is about adult love, that you're gonna do the right thing, because you love yourself. You love your wife. You love your children. You love your mission in life. You're doing this because you want to extend, prolong.

And for me, I love my four children. I never want to live with them. I just don't. I want to...

PEGGY: You mean, live with them, as in, they need to take care of you.

DR AMEN: Absolutely not. I don't want them telling me what to wear, what to eat, taking my driver's license away...

PEGGY: You don't want to be dependent or have them bossing you around.

DR AMEN: No. As if they're paying me back for any sin I have committed. I'm like...

PEGGY: Not going to happen.

DR AMEN: ...I want to be independent.

PEGGY: All right, let's get to the next one. I could talk to you all day just about letter "B", but we'll move on to "R", which is retirement and aging, and that, in and of itself, you consider retirement a risk factor for cognitive decline.

DR AMEN: It is. When you stop learning, your brain starts dying. You need to be engaged. Now, at some point I may retire.

PEGGY: I can't picture that.

DR AMEN: But I want to retire and do something else. I'm going to do something interesting, something that keeps me passionate and engaged – and I am now, with what I do, so I can't imagine not doing that. But that's really critical, new learning. And not doing things you already know how to do.

For example, I know how to write and I know how to teach, so I need to be doing different things that stretch my brain in new and different ways.

A couple of other risk factors under retirement and aging: high ferritin levels. So ferritin is iron storage, and as we age, especially for men, we tend to store more and more iron. It's one of the reasons not to eat a lot of red meat, because it has a lot of iron.

PEGGY: Iron, okay.

DR AMEN: If you have low iron levels, as many women do, red meat's awesome. High iron levels – bad. And the way you decrease it: decrease red meat, decrease red wine (I know people already hate me!)

PEGGY: Decrease red wine?

DR AMEN: Yeah, because red wine...

PEGGY: Did I just hear you say that?

DR AMEN: ...increases the absorption of iron in your diet.

PEGGY: Aw, you just disappointed me. Okay.

DR AMEN: The other way really to decrease your ferritin levels, or your iron storage, is donating blood, which is good for you, and good for other people. Now, there's one other way around it, but I hesitate to mention it... I was at the spice market in Istanbul a couple of years ago, and outside they had leeches for sale. I looked at my wife...

PEGGY: I don't know if you're going to make that sale here today!

DR AMEN: I looked at my wife, and I'm like, "Why are the leeches here?" And she's a nurse, and she said, "It's a health practice, that people bleed themselves in order to keep themselves healthy."

PEGGY: Well, I know that from Victorian novels.

DR AMEN: And my reaction is, "I'm going to the Red Cross."

PEGGY: Yeah. I'm not going to do leeches, like Victorian novels, when they... No.

Okay, "I" is, I believe, inflammation? Am I correct?

DR AMEN: "I" is for inflammation.

PEGGY: Okay, all right.

DR AMEN: It comes from the Latin word, "to set afire." When you have high inflammation in your body, it's as if you have a low-level fire destroying your organs. We measure it with something called "C-reactive protein."

PEGGY: Right.

DR AMEN: Also, your Omega-3 index. If you have low levels of Omega-3's – rampant in this country – you often have high levels of inflammation. We did a study of 200 consecutive patients at the Amen Clinics; 95% of them had low levels of Omega-3 fatty acids.

PEGGY: Wow.

DR AMEN: We just published a new study in *The Journal of Alzheimer's Disease* that showed the effects of high Omega-3 index in your body.

PEGGY: Right.

DR AMEN: Scarlett and Sam were bigger at high levels; low, they were smaller. So you want to make sure you're either eating fish once or twice a week, or taking fish oil to keep your Omega-3s high. And you want to decrease the Omega-6s in your diet, especially the processed corn and soy vegetable oils – not a great thing for inflammation.

PEGGY: We know inflammation is horrible for the brain, but it's horrible for every other part of your body, too. So we'll move on to "G", genetics.

DR AMEN: Genetics. If you have Alzheimer's or a form of dementia in your family, you have a higher risk.

Now, it's not a death sentence. It's a wake-up call. I have heart disease in my family. I have obesity in my family. I don't have heart disease myself, and I don't have obesity. Why? Because I don't engage in the behaviors that are likely to trigger my genetic risk.

The going theory for the causes of Alzheimer's – and there's lots of controversy, you know – asks "Is it beta-amyloid? Is it tau?" You know, these involve buildup of proteins that cause short circuits in the brain. It's controversial at this point.

We know if you have Alzheimer's disease and we give you a drug that clears out the beta-amyloid, it's not going to help you. There have been 2,000 medication trials. It's like, get over it.

PEGGY: And that's been the model, right.

DR AMEN: It's like the Alzheimer's research community has a learning disability. It's like, come on, get over it. You need to be...

PEGGY: "There's a new way to get out the plaque." No, doesn't work.

DR AMEN: So you either need to get rid of it a lot earlier, before the damage occurs... And there are ways to do that. Vitamin D and curcumin have been found to decrease the plaques thought to be responsible for Alzheimer's disease. Blueberries, sage... But you need to be putting these habits into your life when you're young, not when you're...

PEGGY: You're old.

DR AMEN: When you're old. But the "G" of genetics... The whole point of "G" is, don't think of it as a death sentence. Think of it as a wake-up call, and be serious. Green tea is another thing that increases the beta-amyloid plaques.

"H" is so important. It's head trauma, and it's funny, many of the really well-known Alzheimer's researchers don't talk about it. And it's clearly a risk factor.

I did the big NFL study at a time when the NFL was lying, and they were having a problem. We've scanned and treated 200 players, and the level of damage was just awful, and the level of dementia was awful.

But the exciting news is if you've had head trauma, you need to put your brain in a healing environment. And 80% of our players show improvement when they do the right things. So I'm really excited about it.

But don't let your kids play contact sports. It's just not thoughtful when we know your brain is soft, about the consistency of soft butter. Your skull is really hard, and has sharp bony ridges. Your brain runs your life. Damage it, and you actually damage the hardware of your soul. It's a bad idea. We need to be much more thoughtful.

The American Youth Soccer Organization said if you're under 11 you shouldn't be hitting soccer balls with your head. It was a huge positive step, but in my mind, I'm thinking... You don't like 12-year-olds... you don't like 14-year-olds... At what point is it useful to have repetitive hits to the part of your body that is the CEO of your life? It's just not rational. Protect your brain. It's the most important thing.

PEGGY: I was really amazed in your book, in the section on head trauma, you said that with most people who come to you, when you see visible evidence of trauma in their scans, they don't remember that they ever had an injury. And you say, "Did you ever fall off a horse? Were you in a car accident?" They have no memory that something occurred, that you're seeing decades later, showing up in scans, and that's common.

DR AMEN: I mean, it's just unbelievable. Now, they'll eventually tell us about the trauma, but it's like we have to ask them ten times.

I had a patient – one of my NFL players, who was on five Super Bowl teams, Marvin Fleming. He was the starting tight end. And I'm like, "Hey, Marvin (his brain looked awful), did you ever have a brain injury?"

He said, "No." I'm like – and I'm like, "Really?" And he's like, "No, I've never been knocked out. I never got my bell rung." And I'm looking at his brain, and I'm asking, "Well, what about before football?" "Nope."

PEGGY: Nope.

DR AMEN: And then I start with the questions. "Did you ever fall out of a tree? Off a fence? Dive into a shallow pool? Concussions playing sports?" "Nope, nope, nope." "In a car accident?" "Oh, well there was this one time when I was driving from Utah, where I went to college, to Los Angeles. And I got in an accident on a mountain pass, and my car fell 150 feet off a cliff into the river below."

PEGGY: Oh, but I didn't remember to tell you that! That just happened. I didn't think that that might affect my brain.

DR AMEN: It's nuts! And then other people go through windshields of a car, fall out of moving vehicles, fall out of a second story window...

PEGGY: Oh, you hear it all over here. You hear it all.

DR AMEN: And mild traumatic brain injury... There's nothing mild about that. Traumatic brain injury ruins people's lives, and people don't know about it. It's a major cause of depression, suicide, homelessness, and addiction.

PEGGY: Addiction.

DR AMEN: Studies from Toronto – 58% of the homeless men in Toronto and 42% of the homeless women had a significant brain injury before they were homeless. Think it counts?

PEGGY: I think it counts. You know, again, in that section I found something so interesting, you noted that the pituitary gland is located in the skull, right? And that frequently an injury may affect that, which then affects hormonal balance. Did I get that correctly?

DR AMEN: You did, and it's new information. Most people don't know that information.

PEGGY: Yeah, that was new to me.

DR AMEN: In my NFL group, we had to test all their hormones. And you know, here are these big, strapping guys who have testosterone below normal. They have no sex drive, and they're sad, and their memory's no good, and a little testosterone can just be so helpful in that condition.

PEGGY: And that lack of testosterone may have been set off by a head injury.

DR AMEN: Often set up by head trauma.

PEGGY: That's so important.

DR AMEN: So important.

PEGGY: It's so important. I want to mention two things, just to linger on the section for a minute, because you're such an expert, because you see the brain scans of the football players, so you know this in such a deep way.

The two things I think maybe we should talk about are, first, you may very well have had some kind of head injury in the past that's affecting your behavior in negative ways, and you haven't considered that as a possible source of your problem.

And the second one is, Dr. Amen says you can do something about it – that you can make your brain look prettier in the pictures, and feel better if you follow this program, right? Did I say that right?

DR AMEN: 80% of our players showed improvement in as little as two months. You just need to put your brain in a healing environment.

PEGGY: Okay, so that was "H" for head trauma. "T" – toxins.

DR AMEN: "T" is for toxins, one of the sleeper causes of dementia. When I first started looking at brain scans, alcohol – it's just so clear, alcohol is not a health food. It just gives your brain...

PEGGY: Does anybody think it is?

DR AMEN: A lot of people think it is.

PEGGY: Oh.

DR AMEN: The general population, I believe, thinks they should have their two glasses of red wine a day, that it's good for them. Well, according to a study from Johns Hopkins, people who drink every day have smaller brains. And when it comes to your brain, size matters.

PEGGY: Size matters.

DR AMEN: It's the only organ in your body where actually, size really does matter. And I looked at marijuana brains, and you know, it's legal in 26 states – legal in ten states as a treatment for dementia.

I published a study in December in *The Journal of Alzheimer's Disease* on just about 1,000 pot smokers. Virtually every area of their brain was lower, especially the hippocampus. Meaning, the area that dies first in Alzheimer's disease is lower in pot smokers, and from being a psychiatrist for 35 years, I can tell you the most common complaint among pot smokers is their memory's no good.

Then there are other drugs like cocaine and methamphetamines... So that was easy and clear. They're toxic to brain function. You can just see that on the scans.

But then I started seeing toxic scans in people who said they didn't do drugs, and they didn't drink.

PEGGY: Right. It's something else.

DR AMEN: And then I went, "Oh-oh... Mold exposure, carbon monoxide exposure..."

PEGGY: Carbon monoxide?

DR AMEN: Think of firefighters who get exposed to carbon monoxide...

PEGGY: Oh, emergency responders, yeah.

DR AMEN: ...and cyanide... Almost all the firefighters I see have toxic-looking brains.

Same for pilots. When the government, in its wisdom, took lead out of gasoline, they left it in small aircraft fuel. And I'm like, "Why'd you do that?" But you often see the toxicity.

And did you know – I hate this – 60% of the lipstick sold in the United States still has lead in it? I call it "the kiss of death."

PEGGY: Ooh, some of us wear lipstick every day, you know.

DR AMEN: You have to be very careful about who you kiss, and what you put on your lips, because you wear it all day long. It's not a good thing.

And then I was completely horrified. There's a great app – and there are a couple of them that do this – but the one I like is called "Think Dirty." You can scan all of your products like shampoo and body wash and cosmetics and deodorant and hair gel, and so on, and it'll tell you on a scale of one to ten how quickly it's going to kill you, how toxic it is...

PEGGY: You talk pretty straight to us, don't you?

DR AMEN: ...and I literally threw out half my bathroom. I was like, "Oh, my goodness!" So it says things like phthalates, and parabens, and PEGs, and fragrance... Get rid of it – because they're all known endocrine disruptors.

You wonder why the girls are having their menstrual periods earlier and earlier, and why so many men have low testosterone levels. Yes, it could be the head trauma. It could also be the endocrine disruptors they're putting on their bodies without even giving it one thought.

You always want to support the four organs of detoxification. I mean, the big principle with toxins is "limit your exposure."

PEGGY: Okay.

DR AMEN: Right? I mean, buy organics; you don't want to consume pesticides. That should be obvious. Read the labels, and don't buy things that contain toxins. When it comes to personal care products, remember that whatever goes on your body, goes in your body.

Your skin is the largest surface area, and it brings things in. So whatever you put on it goes in it.

Support your kidneys; drink more water. Support your gut; eat more fiber. Support your skin; sweat, either with exercise or taking saunas. A new study from Finland showed people who took the most saunas had the lowest risk of dementia. And support your liver with... I like a supplement called N-acetylcysteine. It helps with detoxification.

And then, eat brassicas, which is a new term for me. I go to a restaurant here in Newport Beach, where I live, and there's something called "brassicas." And I'm like, "What are those?" They're detoxifying vegetables.

PEGGY: Brassicas?

DR AMEN: It's a group of vegetables that includes kale, Brussel sprouts, broccoli, cabbage, cauliflower. And you know, in a little olive oil with salt, they taste awesome.

PEGGY: Cruciferous vegetables.

DR AMEN: It's good for me, and it tastes great, right? And that's the secret to memory rescue with food. It's got to be good for you, but you have to make it taste great.

PEGGY: Yeah, because if it tastes great, you'll eat it. Otherwise, it will remain a good idea that you...

DR AMEN: See, I grew up Catholic, like, "No kidding, cowboy." My mom was serious. I was an altar boy till I was 19, and I'm done with long-suffering. I'm not doing the suffering part.

PEGGY: You want to enjoy.

DR AMEN: I want to love it, but I only will eat things that love me back. I don't love food that doesn't love me. See, I've been in bad relationships in the past. I'm not doing that anymore. I'm not going to love someone who doesn't love me back. I've been there.

PEGGY: Okay.

DR AMEN: It's not fun. It's painful. It's stressful. I'm damn sure not to be in love with Rocky Road ice cream, because it doesn't love me back.

So I'll find sweet treats. Here at Amen Clinics, we actually make a bar called "Brain In Love," and another one called "Brain On Joy," which are sugar-free, dairy-free, gluten-free chocolate sweetened with Stevia and erythritol. Brain On Joy is the coconut one, and they taste awesome. And it's a metaphor, right? I love things that serve my health, not steal my health.

PEGGY: What you're saying harkens back to what you started with, that you have to love your brain.

DR AMEN: Definitely do.

PEGGY: You have to love your brain. You have to decide, "I'm going to fall in love with my brain," if you're not already in love. One thing that helped me fall in love with my brain was your statistic that the brain fires 18 trillion times a second. Did I get that right?

DR AMEN: You did.

PEGGY: I mean, that's pretty exciting.

DR AMEN: It has the storage capacity of six million years of *The Wall Street Journal*, if you take care of it.

PEGGY: If you take care of it. If you love your brain.

DR AMEN: If you love it.

PEGGY: Okay, now we've finished bright in our mnemonic device, and now we're up to "M", which I believe is mental health.

DR AMEN: Mental health issues – rampant among people with memory problems and dementia. We know depression doubles the risk in women and quadruples the risk in men. Also, PTSD, bipolar disorder, schizophrenia, chronic stress, grief... all significantly increase the risk of memory problems. There's a new study on ADHD increasing the risk of a type of dementia called Lewy body dementia.

And what that means to me is you need to manage your mental health. Now, the cool thing is this Bright Minds approach?

PEGGY: Right.

DR AMEN: It's the same approach I use for depression. It's the same approach I use for addictions. It's the same approach I use...

PEGGY: It's healing. It's healing.

DR AMEN: ...for anxiety. It's just a smart approach to your mental and physical well-being. But I also talk about killing the ants, which stands for the "automatic negative thoughts" that steal your happiness and rob you of your mind.

Whenever you feel sad, or mad, or nervous, or out of control, write down what you're thinking, and then talk back to it. Question it. I don't know if you were good talking back to your parents when you were a teenager...

PEGGY: Oh, I was very well behaved.

DR AMEN: I was excellent at talking back to my parents.

PEGGY: Oh, at talking back.

DR AMEN: I was excellent, but no one ever taught me I should talk back to the stupidity that goes on in my own mind.

PEGGY: Good point.

DR AMEN: It's like, you don't have to believe every stupid thought you have. And just some really simple things... Whenever you argue with reality – I learned this from my friend, Byron Katie – whenever you argue with reality, welcome to hell.

PEGGY: Yeah, yeah.

DR AMEN: It's learning to be present in the moment, accept what is, and of course, do the things you can to change it. But mindset is just so important.

And then having a regular stress management practice. I like hypnosis, and self-hypnosis. I practiced it for many years. A lot of people like meditation. There's one I love called "Loving Kindness Meditation."

PEGGY: Yes. I like that. Can you tell us a little bit about that?

DR AMEN: It's purposeful thinking, if you will. It starts with loving yourself. "May I be happy... may I be healthy... may I be safe." So it consists of coming up with little mantras. You do it for a minute for yourself. You just repeat that. And then to someone you're grateful for: "May Peggy be happy... may Peggy be healthy... may Peggy be safe."

PEGGY: Thank you.

DR AMEN: And then you repeat it for someone you're sort of neutral on, and then someone you just don't like, someone you're having a hard time with.

PEGGY: Okay, okay.

DR AMEN: And I've had plenty of critics...

PEGGY: You have a full supply.

DR AMEN: ...so I'm happy to get them in on the fun. And then you do it to the whole world, and it is such positive directed emotion and tension that it's been found to decrease the stress found in soldiers who had PTSD. It's been found to decrease headaches. It's been found to decrease cortisol. And it's simple. Five minutes a day.

PEGGY: It's simple. It's not a medication.

DR AMEN: Twenty minutes a day. There's no meds involved with it. And people go, "Well, if I have depression, does that mean medication?" And it's like this practice is head-to-head against medication.

Saffron has been found to be equally effective. I'm a huge fan of saffron.

PEGGY: Of saffron.

DR AMEN: There are so many reasons.

PEGGY: Good.

DR AMEN: Exercise has been found to be equally effective, if you can get people to do it. Omega-3 fatty acids, equally effective in killing the ants, those automatic negative thoughts, learning how not to believe every stupid thought you have.

PEGGY: A behavioral approach...

DR AMEN: Make a thinking adjustment. And before we do meds, why don't we do saffron, and exercise, Omega-3 fatty acids, and let me teach you how to kill the ants.

PEGGY: Because you're such an expert on brain scans, what brains look like – just to stay with mental health for a minute – can you look at a brain and say, "This is PTSD. This is borderline. This is schizophrenia. This is depression..." I mean, do the scans look different?

DR AMEN: They do, but it's important to know that depression's not one thing.

PEGGY: Right.

DR AMEN: I wrote a book about that. It's seven different things in the brain. So I can say, "This is a brain that's prone to depression, that's likely to respond to this treatment."

I published a big study on 21,000 people showing we could distinguish traumatic brain injury from PTSD – emotional trauma from physical trauma – with high levels of accuracy.

But I think one of the big principles that underlie our work is that all psychiatric illnesses – all of them – are not single or simple disorders. They all have multiple types, which is why imaging didn't catch on when I got excited about it in the early 90s.

PEGGY: Right.

DR AMEN: Because the researchers were going, "Oh, what's the pattern with major depression?" And I was going, "There's never going to be one, because not everybody responds to Prozac." I can tell if someone's depressed, right? I can talk to somebody for 20 minutes and I know whether or not they're depressed. What I don't know is what's going on in their brains.

PEGGY: What's making that happen.

DR AMEN: It's really a unique fingerprint in your brain for depression. So what's Peggy's depression? Is her brain busy? Is it cold, low in activity? Is it one side or the other side of her brain? So I know what to do, rather than, "Oh, this scan says you're depressed."

PEGGY: Okay. Moving along in our mnemonic, we're back to "I", another "I".

DR AMEN: "I" number two, because it has two things. It has immunity and infections.

PEGGY: Oh, it's a double "I".

DR AMEN: It's a double "I" – very important. Autoimmune disorders like rheumatoid arthritis, MS, and asthma have been associated with memory problems, a higher risk for memory problems. And infections are a major cause of dementia, and still not really well known.

PEGGY: I wanted to talk to you about that for a minute. Several doctors I've spoken to have really emphasized Lyme disease, this epidemic, which then can bring on cognitive problems. But you talk about a lot of other ones that aren't as well known, other viruses, parasites from your pet. You go into a whole bunch of things.

DR AMEN: Toxoplasmosis, right.

PEGGY: Yes, yes. Epstein-Barr... Tell us about all these horrible things that we may not be thinking about.

DR AMEN: I think the big issue is, if you have memory problems and they're not getting better with simple things...

... somebody should do an infectious disease panel to make sure you're not at war with some invader, like toxoplasmosis that comes from cat feces, or Lyme. Kris Kristofferson was diagnosed with Alzheimer's, and actually was found to have Lyme by one of our doctors, and was put on an antibiotic and hyperbaric oxygen. He got brought back, and he's touring again.

Herpes is another one. It's very common, and if you have genital herpes, or you have cold sores, it increases your risk of significant memory problems by 20%. And you know, that affects a third of the population.

PEGGY: Oh, really?

DR AMEN: Really.

PEGGY: Ooh.

DR AMEN: I tell my kids, "Always be careful who you sleep with, because actually, some of their genetic material is going to be mixing with yours." So it's another reason...

PEGGY: Most people's parents do not put it that way, do they? It might be a good thing if people understood that a little more. Okay, so it's ...

DR AMEN: So you want to boost your immune system. How do you do that?

PEGGY: How do you do it?

DR AMEN: Gut health, because you know, the biggest immunity you have is in your gut. Probiotics can help. Also, measure and optimize your vitamin D level. 67% of the population in the U.S. is low in vitamin D, often dangerously low. Normal is between 30 and 100. Optimal, I think, is between 50 and 100.

They did a study at UC San Diego. They looked at people whose D levels were about 40, and people who were below 20. The people who were below 20 had 2.2 times the risk of cancer. By the way, cancer's going to steal your brain because of the stress and the chemotherapy.

PEGGY: Yeah, yeah, yeah.

DR AMEN: Right? So how simple is it just to get a blood test for 25 hydroxy vitamin D. Measure your level and then take steps to get it high. And if you live in New York, where the sun's not out for a long time, you should probably be taking 5,000 units of vitamin D a day. But you know, rather than take that number, ask, "What's your level, and what do you need?"

I live in Southern California. The sun is out 330 days a year here. When I first tested my level, it was 17. I was horrified, and I was hungry all the time. I tried to lose weight in every way you can imagine. When vitamin D is low, the hormone leptin that tells your brain you're not hungry anymore doesn't work.

PEGGY: The appetite suppressant.

DR AMEN: And when I started on vitamin D, my appetite went away. I dropped something like 20 pounds. And I did the right things.

PEGGY: That's the greatest diet ever – take vitamin D.

DR AMEN: Take vitamin D.

PEGGY: I love that diet.

DR AMEN: And love your brain.

PEGGY: Love your brain. Love your brain. Okay, that was a very important letter, "I". Okay, we are doing MINDS... "N" – neuro-hormonal deficiencies. See, I remember. It's a good mnemonic device.

DR AMEN: See? The mnemonic works.

PEGGY: I got it, I got it.

DR AMEN: And you're petting your seahorses. You're being nice to them. You're loving them.

PEGGY: I have very active seahorses, you'll be happy to know.

DR AMEN: So neuro-hormone is just absolutely critical. These hormones are like Miracle Gro for your brain. And when hormones are low, Scarlett and Sam, our seahorses, wither and get smaller, and can die. So you need to measure, for women, their estrogen and progesterone levels; for everybody, their thyroid, DHEA, and testosterone. And I actually don't want them normal. I want them optimal.

PEGGY: Optimal.

DR AMEN: Which usually means around 70 to 100% of high normal. I don't like above normal, especially for testosterone, because if you go above normal, you'll get to be a super guy, which means you'll have a crazy sex drive and have no empathy, which is the prescription for divorce, so...

PEGGY: Oh, we certainly don't want that.

DR AMEN: You don't want that. But at the same time, you want it high enough that you have energy, and motivation, and...

PEGGY: The good drive.

DR AMEN: ...your mood is good, and your libido is healthy.

PEGGY: Yes. And I think you mentioned that you have found that low thyroid is so often correlated with depression.

DR AMEN: Depression and dementia. And what we see is really low blood flow on the scans.

My daughter had a great second-grade teacher, loved her. And she came to me one day and said, "I'm in a Master's program, and I cannot think. Can you help me?" The first thing I did, besides scan her, was to order a battery of tests, and I found a thyroid disorder – she had Hashimoto's thyroiditis.

PEGGY: Oh!

DR AMEN: And she'd seen her primary care doctor...

PEGGY: And he hadn't found it.

DR AMEN: And the only thing he'd ordered was a TSH test, rather than the whole thyroid panel. So I ordered thyroid antibodies, and her body was attacking her thyroid gland. After getting that treated, she went on and got her Master's, and she felt so much happier.

PEGGY: Well, I think one thing we're learning from what you're telling us is there's more tests that you can do. There's more information available to help you pinpoint what's bothering you, the major source of it.

DR AMEN: Right, so which of these 11 risk factors do you have that you need to attack? I mean, ultimately, there's something simple to do for each one of them, like "B" is exercise for blood flow; the solution for retirement and aging is to be engaged and learn new things; "I" is inflammation: take Omega-3 fatty acids, or eat more fish; "G" – genetics. Have it in your family? You've got to be serious. "H" is head trauma – protect your brain. "T" is toxins – don't put anything toxic on your body. You know, get the app, "Think Dirty, " and scan your stuff. "M" – mental health – loving kindness meditation, not believing every stupid thought you have, stress management practices... All of these things are good for all of us, no matter what our age.

And "D" is diabesity.

PEGGY: Diabesity.

DR AMEN: Which is a combination of diabetes and obesity. I published two studies that showed as your weight goes up, the actual physical size and function of your brain goes down.

PEGGY: So your brain gets smaller.

DR AMEN: Your brain gets smaller.

PEGGY: As you get fatter, your brain gets smaller – bad, very bad.

DR AMEN: Dinosaur syndrome – big body, little brain.

PEGGY: Bad.

DR AMEN: You're going to become extinct.

PEGGY: Well, all...

DR AMEN: So bad thing.

PEGGY: Bad. All these things you've told us are going to help us fight diabesity. We know exercise. You've told us to eat properly. You've told us to take vitamin D, which is going to activate the hormone that tells us, "You're full. You don't need any more..." So you've addressed it so many ways.

DR AMEN: None of this is hard, but now we've got to get the food right, because that's how you get diabesity under control. And basically, the principle is "Kill the sugar before it kills you." It's kill the sugar and the foods that turn to sugar – bread, pasta, potatoes, and rice – because they're high glycemic.

I wrote a book called *The Brain Warrior's Way* with my wife, and we make the argument that ISIS has nothing on our food industry.

PEGGY: Oh, man.

DR AMEN: That the real weapons of mass destruction are highly-processed, pesticide-sprayed, high glycemic, low fiber, food-like substances stored in plasticized containers. That two-thirds of Americans are overweight.

PEGGY: Two-thirds. That's stunning.

DR AMEN: One-third to 40% of us are obese. It's the biggest brain drain in the history of the United States, and we're doing to ourselves. It's just nuts. We need to do better. And I think of calories like money: You overspend – you're going to go bankrupt.

I actually like going to places where they have calories on the menu, because if I don't know what's in it, I'm not eating it. Right? I'd never buy something I wouldn't know the cost to it, but also all calories are not the same, right? You want to go with high-quality...

PEGGY: Yes, high quality, nutrient-dense.

DR AMEN: ...nutrient-dense... But you know, we have to stop lying to ourselves. Our obesity epidemic, we're not going to be able to pay for, because the side effects with diabetes, and cancer, heart disease and dementia...

PEGGY: And dementia, which is so costly.

DR AMEN: It's not okay.

PEGGY: So costly.

DR AMEN: That goes back to Chloe's game: whatever I'm getting today, is it good for my brain, or bad for it?

PEGGY: "S" is for sleep – we've got to sleep.

DR AMEN: It's just absolutely critical.

PEGGY: We've got to sleep.

DR AMEN: When you sleep, your brain cleans and washes itself. So if you don't get seven hours at night, the cleanup crew doesn't have enough time to clean up the mess that you made during the day.

PEGGY: That's right.

DR AMEN: And less than seven hours is associated with low blood flow to your brain.

PEGGY: I like that you said that, because that takes us back to the beginning, the low blood flow, you know?

DR AMEN: And if you have low blood flow to your frontal lobes, that means more bad decisions.

PEGGY: More bad decisions, more stress, more everything. It all connects – everything connects with everything else. The program is really coherent. It's really 360 degrees.

DR AMEN: Right, and sleep apnea triples your risk of Alzheimer's disease, because it's an oxygen debt state, and your brain is the most oxygen-hungry organ in your body. And so in order to have a bright mind...

PEGGY: A bright mind.

DR AMEN: You have to attack all the risk factors.

PEGGY: Now we've been through the program. I just want to give people a little information. You've got some extra tricks up your sleeve that most people don't know about that you mentioned...

... like hyperbaric oxygen treatment, and another one. I think it was transcranial stimulation, or something. You have some good tricks, and most people don't know about them, and their doctors may not know about them.

DR AMEN: I'm a huge fan of hyperbaric oxygen, going in a chamber and getting more oxygen under pressure. I've seen it boost blood flow to the brain. I published a study on soldiers showing remarkable increased blood flow, with no side effects, simple to do. Even the home hyperbaric oxygen chambers that don't have as much pressure have been found to be helpful.

Transcranial magnetic stimulation is classically thought of as a treatment for depression, but there's also been studies on memory and dementia showing it can be helpful. Also, neuro-feedback, another treatment shown to be helpful, is super simple. Audiovisual stimulation, glasses and headphones that give you lights and sounds at certain frequencies to help optimize brain function.

PEGGY: I think a lot of people aren't aware that there are these extra tools, and it's important that they know. You know, you shouldn't give up. You shouldn't give up. There might be...

DR AMEN: Lots of things to do.

PEGGY: Yeah, there might be this thing that works.

DR AMEN: So – know what your risk factors are, attack those first, and then try to put the simple things from all of the risk factors in place.

PEGGY: I just have one last question, because we've got through the program, and it's great that we got through it all. I just want you to speculate: what do you think our brains are going to be like in ten years or so, as we age? Because you point out that all these devices that we have are actually changing our attention span, you said... that humans now have an eight-second attention span, and goldfish have a nine-second one, so we're underperforming goldfish.

DR AMEN: Right. They don't have smartphones. They don't have dumb phones. I guess that's the way to put it.

PEGGY: Yeah. How's this all... how are we going to age with this kind of stimulation that we have?

DR AMEN: Well, it's not going to go away, so we have to make peace with it, and we need to make sure we take breaks from it. But, I mean, the study was from Microsoft, online, the human attention span is eight seconds.

PEGGY: Eight seconds.

DR AMEN: And in 2000 it was 12 seconds. So we've lost a third of our attention span in a very short period of time.

PEGGY: That is stunning.

DR AMEN: Hopefully, the scientists you're talking to or people like me will educate people to take better care of their brains.

PEGGY: I love that, and that's the whole... Give us the parting message. I think you just did, but...

DR AMEN: Well, the message of my life is: you're not stuck with the brain you have. You can make it better, even if you've been bad to it. You just have to put it in a healing environment.

PEGGY: Thank you so much, Dr. Amen. I so appreciate it, and thank you so much for watching. I hope you learned a lot from Dr. Amen, and I hope you read his book, *Memory Rescue,* because it really has so much great information that you heard today, and much, much more. So here's to loving your brain.

Interview with Dr. Michael Breus, Ph.D., Clinical Psychologist

PEGGY: Hello, I'm Peggy Sarlin, and today I'm speaking with Dr. Michael Breus in Manhattan Beach, California. Dr. Breus is going to tell us how you can improve your memory by improving your sleep.

Dr. Breus is a nationally-recognized expert on sleep. He's appeared many times on "Dr. Oz," and "Oprah," and "The View," and he's written best-selling books on sleep. So welcome, Dr. Breus.

DR BREUS: Thanks for having me, Peggy. I'm super excited to be here. I think this is a really important topic, and I'm ready to dive right in.

PEGGY: So let me ask you... You have developed a completely new approach to maximize mental energy by working with your body's natural rhythms to get a good night's sleep. Tell us about that.

DR BREUS: That's correct. My theory is called "The Power of When." Most of the time when you're thinking about how to help yourself have more energy, you're learning about what to do, or how to do it. But nobody's ever telling you *when* to do it.

If you remember, everybody's got an internal biological clock called their "circadian rhythm." And it turns out there's three or four different circadian rhythms out there.

Once you know what that circadian rhythm is, you can actually figure out the exact right time of day to do whatever it is you want to do, whether it's read a book... get new information... have a cup of coffee... go for a run... have some mental clarity... be creative... sell... buy. Whatever it is you want to do, there are actually specific times in your biological rhythm when you're better at it, and I've figured out a way to identify them.

PEGGY: That sounds completely new, so I want to try to understand it. The first thing you're saying – help me understand – is that each person is born with an innate circadian rhythm the same way we have a blood type, an innate blood type? Is that an analogy, or...?

DR BREUS: Yes, that's a great analogy *except*...

PEGGY: Except.

DR BREUS: Here's one of the things: We're all genetically predisposed to have a particular circadian rhythm once we reach adulthood. But that circadian rhythm shifts around quite a bit when we're younger.

When we have babies, babies have much longer sleep cycles. Then when you get to adolescence you have a tendency to stay up late and sleep late. But once we hit the 18, 19, 20-year-old stage, roughly speaking, our circadian rhythm is pretty much locked and loaded... until we hit kind of our senior stages, where it has a tendency to dial back, and we want to go to bed earlier and wake up earlier.

Once we know which one of those age ranges you're in, we can actually section that off to learn whether you could be a little bit ahead or a little bit behind.

Many people have heard of something called an "early bird," – right? – or a "night owl." So once you know if you're an early bird, a night owl, something in between, or somebody who's not such a great sleeper... once you've figured that part out, that's when you can dial it in and know exactly what time of day things are working.

But it is a lot like a blood type. It just happens to change a little bit until you get to be an adult.

PEGGY: So let's talk about seniors, because we want to talk about improving memory.

DR BREUS: Sure.

PEGGY: And once you get to be a senior you may have senior moments.

DR BREUS: Sure.

PEGGY: You may have brain fog, not feel so sharp. So does that mean your circadian rhythm has changed, or what? Help us understand.

DR BREUS: Sure. It's interesting. As we get older our circadian rhythm has a tendency to go backwards. As a result, we want to go to bed earlier and wake up earlier, which means there are certain times of the day that it's better for us to have information than others.

As an example, if you're going to read a book and your circadian rhythm is early as you get older, when's the best time to potentially read a book? Well, it turns out that the earlier part of the morning is probably the best time for several reasons.

Number one, the level of melatonin (which, remember, is the key that starts the engine for sleep) is off so you don't have melatonin making you feel that brain fogginess – which, by the way, is one of the reasons why you do. Number two is you hopefully by that point have had some input as far as energy is concerned, right? I mean, a little bit of nutrition, something to get the brain going. But you haven't gotten to the point where you've exhausted that resource or that nutrition.

So as an example, if you're waking up at 5:30, 6:00, when should you read a book? You should probably start reading a book, or an article, or a newspaper or something like that within 90-120 minutes of waking up, so somewhere between an hour and a half and two hours of waking up is going to be your prime time to receive new information.

PEGGY: Okay, let's just stop there. So by reading a book – I mean, I might read a book to relax and fall asleep.

DR BREUS: Sure.

PEGGY: But by "reading a book" you mean this is the time when your brain is most receptive to processing new information.

DR BREUS: Exactly, yes. That's a perfect way to think about it.

PEGGY: Okay.

DR BREUS: Absolutely.

PEGGY: So I've woken up early and naturally. I've woken up. The sunlight has woken me up.

DR BREUS: Right.

PEGGY: Because I'm older now, and I'm... okay.

DR BREUS: Absolutely.

PEGGY: And now what do I do? Now, when's my best time to eat?

DR BREUS: The first thing you do when you wake up early is you hydrate, okay? You want to drink either a glass or a bottle of water as quickly as you can. Why? Because remember, during your sleep you've actually breathed out almost a liter of fluid. So we don't want you to get dehydrated.

Also, if you're on medication there are certain medications that can give you a dry mouth, things like that. So go ahead and hydrate first.

Second thing you want to do is, if the sun is up, go outside and get some sunlight. We know that direct sunlight helps turn off that melatonin pump and reset the circadian clock. So you do those two things at first.

Then you have your nutrition. Personally, I like to do a shake or some kind of smoothie, or something like that. That way I can get in a good amount of protein early in the morning, because you want to start your day off with that kind of fuel in your tank.

You need to be careful. You don't want to have a whole lot of carbohydrates in the morning. It turns out carbohydrates make you feel sleepy because they elevate levels of serotonin. We actually want protein in your system because that's going to get you going.

Once you've done those three things – hydration, sunlight and nutrition – that's the time that you're going to want to go and get some new information.

PEGGY: And use your brain. And when we're talking about sunlight, we also are talking about exercise.

DR BREUS: That's a great point.

PEGGY: For instance, we're talking about taking a walk.

DR BREUS: Absolutely.

PEGGY: Ten minutes in the morning.

DR BREUS: Yeah... walk the family dog... go down to the mailbox – whatever it is – just walk around the block a couple of times – absolutely that is going to be a good idea.

Now, though, when you're looking at information though, and you're trying to do an analysis, whether it's pay your bills, or learn something new, or write a letter, those types of things, that's one kind of information. But there's also a different kind of information that sometimes people are looking at, and that's more creative.

So what's a good time to be creative? The opposite, believe it or not. It's better for people to be creative in the later afternoon when you're a little bit more tired, because your analytical side is now starting to shut down, but your creative side is starting to kick in.

As an example, if you like to paint, are an artist or a poet... or whatever it is you like to do, that's a great time, sort of the middle afternoon. Try to avoid the middle afternoon nap if you can, because that would be a perfect time to be really creative.

PEGGY: Let's go back to that morning walk.

DR BREUS: Alright.

PEGGY: I'm trying to understand, because we're talking about setting our circadian rhythm.

DR BREUS: Right.

PEGGY: Let's go back to this concept of taking a walk in the morning and exposing your eyes to morning light. Is there something about the quality of the light itself in the morning, as opposed to the light at dusk that is going to work with your body?

DR BREUS: Natural light is natural light, so you'll get the specific wavelength, 460 nanometers of light. That's the blue light that's in the light spectrum, which has the ability to turn off that melatonin pump and help give you energy.

So it doesn't necessarily matter, the morning light versus the evening light. What matters is the timing of the light. So getting that light in the morning helps reset that circadian clock, and that's going to be one of the big things.

A lot of patients turn to me and they say, "You know, I feel like I've got brain fog," right?

PEGGY: Yes.

DR BREUS: And they feel like, "Oh my gosh, something's going on with me. What's happening here?" A lot of times what's going on is you're not waking up with your circadian rhythm.

So as an example, I have a lot of patients who say, "Well, I don't want to get up at 5:30 in the morning. Even though my brain wakes me up and I wake up, I'm just going to lie there and kind of hit the snooze button, or doze in and doze out."

It turns out that's not the best idea because what that ends up doing is basically telling your brain it's okay to continue to produce melatonin – and it does. And then when you really have to wake up you feel tired and sluggish, and you don't really have that level of energy you're looking for. So it's about consistency, and it's about listening to your body.

PEGGY: Let's go back to the patient who wakes up at 5:30.

DR BREUS: Okay.

PEGGY: If they wake up, should they get up? Is that it?

DR BREUS: Absolutely.

PEGGY: You're telling us, once you're up, you're up.

DR BREUS: What I'm telling you is once you've gotten an amount of sleep and you have a consistent wake-up time, respect the consistent wake-up time. Right?

A lot of people who might be watching this interview could be retired or not have a full-time position that they have to wake up to every morning. What I suggest to people is pick a wake-up time, just like you pick a bedtime, and stick to it.

The more consistent you are, the better you're going to be able to perform, and the better my system will actually work.

If you wake up at the same time and go to bed at the same time, you'll know what your circadian rhythm is because your body will shift one way or another and allow you to do that. Once you've figured that part out, then you can go to the specific activities like going for a walk in the morning, which I do recommend.

PEGGY: So let's go back to that 5:30 in the morning.

DR BREUS: Yup.

PEGGY: Let's say I have said to myself, "Okay, I'm going to go to bed at ten o'clock every night, and I'm going to wake up at six every day."

DR BREUS: Okay.

PEGGY: Now I'm waking up at 5:00 or 5:30, so what should I do?

DR BREUS: If you wake up at 5:30, your brain is done. You don't need any more sleep. Go ahead and get up.

PEGGY: That's it?

DR BREUS: Absolutely.

PEGGY: Yeah, okay. Three in the morning?

DR BREUS: Three in the morning's a little bit different. If you're waking at three in the morning, you have to look at what time you went to sleep, and also, it doesn't make a whole lot of sense to wake up at three in the morning.

What I find with a lot of my patients who wake up at three is that they went to bed at eight.

PEGGY: Oh.

DR BREUS: So they're really getting seven hours of sleep.

PEGGY: But you're talking about older people, they may need to go to the bathroom.

DR BREUS: They may wake up to go to the bathroom. That's certainly one of the things that happens. But what I find with some of my seniors is that their day is over by 7:30, 8:00. They're bored. There's not anything else for them to do, and so they end up in the bedroom. They watch a little television and then they fall asleep, so they actually perpetuate the issue by not staying up.

I used to have a treatment I called "The Jay Leno Treatment." I would tell people, "Stay up and watch Jay Leno's monologue," and...

PEGGY: They'd have to stay up a long time now!

DR BREUS: Now, because he's not on anymore, I know. But maybe it's the Jimmy Fallon show, I don't know. But you know what I'm talking about. If you stay up a little bit later, believe it or not – I know this sounds very counterintuitive – but if you stay up a little bit later you'll actually sleep a little bit better.

PEGGY: OK, so take us through. Our goal now is that you're telling us when we should be doing certain things – you're structuring our day for maximum mental efficiency.

DR BREUS: Absolutely. Exactly.

PEGGY: Take us through the morning. Now we've woken up. We've hydrated.

DR BREUS: We've hydrated.

PEGGY: We've had a glass of water.

DR BREUS: Right. We've gotten some sunlight, we've gotten our nutrition.

PEGGY: We've had some protein.

DR BREUS: We've had some protein. Hopefully, with our sunlight, we might even have gotten a little bit of exercise, so now what do we do?

There's a lot of different activities you can do in the morning, especially because that's probably going to be your most clear time. So that's when I would say you want to have activities that are going to require a lot of detail work. Whether it's paying bills, or writing letters, or doing research, or reading for a purpose – not reading for pleasure, per se, but reading for a purpose.

PEGGY: We're talking about focus.

DR BREUS: Exactly.

PEGGY: Let's talk about, what are the mental characteristics? You know, there's focus, there's processing, there's speed...

DR BREUS: Right.

PEGGY: Take us through some of the different aspects of getting stuff done.

DR BREUS: Sure. When you look at something like focus – focus is one of those things that's actually going to happen early in your circadian cycle, whereas creativity is going to happen later in your circadian cycle, and that has to do with hormones.

What happens is, when you wake up in the morning your cortisol level is at its highest point, because that's what helps you wake up, and then it slowly starts to drift down throughout the day, right? Melatonin is lowest in the morning, and it slowly starts to gain during the day.

So the point when those two cross is when you pop over to the other side, and that's when you're more creative. It doesn't mean that you can't still do different activities. It just means you're going to be more relaxed. You're not going to be as focused. You're not going to be as analytical.

You're going to be more, "I'm going to go with the flow," or "I'm going to be more creative," or "I'm going to get more involved in a new activity."

PEGGY: So how many hours of good focus time does our body naturally give us?

DR BREUS: Well, it gives it to us in chunks. So what I would say is it's very difficult to focus for anything longer than about 45-55 minutes without taking a break, because your eyes get tired. Your brain gets tired. Fatigue sets in.

And this is all assuming a normal, healthy adult, as opposed to maybe somebody out there who's got high blood pressure, or who may have a cognitive dysfunction, or something like that, because that can disrupt things quite a bit. But I would say you've got 45-50 minutes of heavy focus, then rehydrate.

PEGGY: Rehydrate.

DR BREUS: I'm a big hydration guy, but I promise you, it really works. Also, walk outside. Get a little bit more sunlight.

PEGGY: Outside some more.

DR BREUS: Absolutely.

PEGGY: Okay, so we want to keep – It's almost like nourishment.

DR BREUS: It is. There's no question. The human form thrives with sunlight. You know, a lot of times we're locking ourselves into offices all day, and we're getting artificial light, and there's nothing better for you than natural sunlight.

Now, of course, if it's winter and you're in New York City, it might not be so easy to walk outside during the wintertime. But then just move your chair over to a window so you're able to get some of that sunlight, or open a window for a brief period of time.

Also air quality – it turns out to be a big thing as well. When you're cooped up inside and the heat is running on and on, you're not getting really good, fresh air. That's also going to be a real big help for you as well.

PEGGY: This is like our grandparents' wisdom: Go outside and get some fresh air! Working with the body.

DR BREUS: Yes, but it's true. The data's really consistent on it.

One of the other things I have a lot of people do is deep breathing exercises just before lunch. So many, many people out there are very shallow breathers, or they're too big a breather, right? A big breather takes in this big volume of air, and then they kind of breathe in and breathe out.

What you really want is a nice, consistent breath that's kind of lasting all day. But a lot of times we forget to breathe. I know that sounds sort of crazy, but it's true. You get so involved, and you all of a sudden notice, "Oh, my gosh, I'm not breathing right now."

What you really want to do right before lunch is what's called "diaphragmatic breathing." So you want to really breathe in to be able to fill your chest up, right? And then you hold it for a couple or three seconds, and then you breathe out, and you really let that come out.

PEGGY: Show us. Give us a diaphragmatic breath.

DR BREUS: You would go, "In... two... three... four...; Hold it... two... three... four...; and then out... two... three... four." You would do that about five or ten times. What it does is it re-centers you. It re-focuses you. It makes you right where you want to be. Like, you can even tell a difference in my voice...

PEGGY: Yeah, I noticed.

DR BREUS: ...after just doing that.

PEGGY: Yeah.

DR BREUS: Right? Is it really –

PEGGY: You sound mellow.

DR BREUS: Yeah, it really brings you into a good space. Then, of course, you're going to have a good, healthy lunch, depending upon what you want that to be. That's where you can have, probably, the bulk of your carbohydrates, by the way – at lunch. Because remember, carbohydrates can make you feel sleepy, but you also are going to need some energy to pull you through the rest of the day, and the protein you had at breakfast has probably worn off by lunchtime or so.

After you've had a good, nutritious lunch, there's an issue that's going to come up. Between one and three in the afternoon most people feel sleepy.

PEGGY: Most people.

DR BREUS: They do. And that's actually evolutionary, believe it or not. If you go into Latin American countries, what do most people do during one and three?

PEGGY: Siesta.

DR BREUS: Siesta, right? So there's an evolution there. What really is going on is that your biology, your core body temperature has a small dip between one and three in the afternoon, and that causes a release of melatonin, which makes you feel sleepy.

So if you want to avoid that dip, and avoid taking a nap and ending up on the couch for 90 minutes, go outside again.

PEGGY: Aha!

DR BREUS: Sunlight stops the production of melatonin. The thing I think that's important for people to realize, not just from a circadian standpoint, but from an overall brain health standpoint, is the role of light is medicine.

Light has a dramatic effect on you, and then once you understand how light can have an effect on you and your body, you can do a lot of really interesting things with it to allow you to be more alert, or to allow you to fall asleep, whatever you choose.

PEGGY: I think most of us don't appreciate that enough. For most of us, our lives are very much cooped inside.

DR BREUS: Yes, exactly.

PEGGY: And there's all this healing right outside our door that we can access. So you are recommending that we build cycles into our day of going outside and getting even just a few minutes of fresh air.

DR BREUS: Right, exactly. Yeah.

PEGGY: It may not be so easy for people working nine to five jobs and so forth, but...

DR BREUS: But they do get breaks, right?

PEGGY: They do get breaks.

DR BREUS: So what I oftentimes tell people is, "Hey, look, if you've got a break going on, then go outside and just walk around the block. Or if you can't even go outside but you want to get a little bit of energy, walk up and down the stairs a couple of times. Just get the blood flowing." It turns out that sitting for too long ain't good.

PEGGY: Sitting for too long is not good, and of course, we're sitting at our desk all day, most of us. So there you go.

DR BREUS: Right, exactly. And so it's really about movement.

The second big point, aside from the fact that light is medicine, is that movement is medicine. When you look at Tai Chi as an example, it's not like they're exercising, but the sheer movement and flow of the body actually helps with circulation, and circulation is your friend because circulation moves resources from one part of the body to another.

So as your body is consuming resources and needing it, if you don't move, your body doesn't flow. If your body doesn't flow, you don't get the resources that you want.

So really, standing up every 50-55 minutes really stretching, breathing, all of these things... And I know they sound basic, but honestly, they're simple to do and they have a tremendous effect if you do them on a consistent basis.

PEGGY: So when you say "breathing," going back to that diaphragmatic breathing that you spoke to us about before, the Tai Chi – quite a few doctors whom I've spoken to have recommended Tai Chi for brain health.

DR BREUS: Yes.

PEGGY: And for seniors, in particular, it's gentle. And that's something you could even do at your office desk.

DR BREUS: Exactly.

PEGGY: But it's crossing the meridians that's the healing motion.

DR BREUS: Right. Exactly. You know, many people don't really understand Tai Chi, but it's not like you have to study it in China for 20 years to be able to do it. That's the good news, right, is you have a midline, or your meridian, and as you cross the meridian, you open up muscles and you allow those muscles to breathe, if you will.

And what you're really doing is you're allowing for better circulation. So, again, it about the distribution of vitamins, nutrients, minerals – all those things need to get to the places they need to go. And when you're sitting, you're blocking the river, if you will, and you need to get the river flowing.

PEGGY: Well, you know, when you talked about that sleepy time in the afternoon, the sluggish feeling, it seems like you're recommending the perfect solution, which is getting that river flowing. If you feel sluggish – get it circulating.

DR BREUS: Exactly. And you know, when people are out there and they're saying, "Oh, my gosh, I'm having a senior moment," or "I'm having brain fog," or something like that, take a look back. Are you well hydrated? Did you sleep well? Have you moved today?

PEGGY: Yes.

DR BREUS: Right? Those are three things I would ask people to do on a fairly regular basis. And the way you know if you slept well? Does your partner say that you snore? Do you wake up feeling refreshed? Has anybody ever seen you stop breathing in your sleep?

Those are signs of something called "sleep apnea" which affects the quality of sleep. So you might have slept for seven hours, but if it wasn't a good seven hours, you're not going to feel too well, and that's where brain fog is going to come in.

PEGGY: So if you wake up... you've put in the time... you've been in the bed, but you feel exhausted, a potential explanation is sleep apnea?

DR BREUS: Absolutely. Remember, sleep is not just a quantity issue; it's a quality issue as well. And I have lots of patients say to me, "Oh, Dr. Breus, I sleep eight hours, but gosh, I'm exhausted all day." Well, my question is, are they eight good hours?

PEGGY: Well, okay, let's get to sleep. Let's keep going through the day.

DR BREUS: Uh huh.

PEGGY: So right now we have powered our way through our sluggish period.

DR BREUS: Exactly.

PEGGY: We've gotten up at our desk. We've stretched, done some exercises. We've had some more water... Let me ask you a question: Suppose I'm feeling forgetful. I can't remember, did I put my glasses here or there, or the other...? At that moment, would it be a good idea to have some water, to do some deep breathing?

DR BREUS: It would be.

PEGGY: I mean, to put it into place right then, at that moment?

DR BREUS: Absolutely. We know that as you become dehydrated, or as your breathing is too shallow, what you're doing is you're depleting your body of those resources that it needs, and that's what's causing the brain fog, in a lot of cases.

Now, I'm not suggesting that there aren't other reasons for brain fog, that there aren't neurochemical reasons and all that. But what I'm saying is, from a more holistic approach, when you walk into someplace and you can't find your glasses... slow down for a second. Breathe.

PEGGY: Right. Breathe. Diaphragmatic breathing.

DR BREUS: Diaphragmatic breathing, get some water, relax for a second and allow yourself the time to remember. And you will remember.

PEGGY: Give the file time to download.

DR BREUS: Yeah, exactly.

PEGGY: Just help it out a little bit.

DR BREUS: Exactly.

PEGGY: Okay, we're now at three in the afternoon. We've powered our way through our siesta. We didn't need it.

DR BREUS: Right, we don't – yup.

PEGGY: Now what do we do?

DR BREUS: In a lot of cases, especially from a senior standpoint, we're really in the last third of our day at that point. So at that point – it's not necessarily a bad idea – If you didn't have time to exercise in the morning, that might not be a bad time for you to exercise.

This is actually your more creative period of time, after about three in the afternoon, believe it or not. And so what's the time to do creative activities? Brainstorming about new, fun things that you want to try... or thinking about family, calling family members, reconnecting in that way, when you're not as analytical, but more emotional, more creative.

That's a great time to call some family member you haven't talked to in a little while, or have that discussion with your spouse, or something along those lines because you've got some time to do that.

Now, if you're at work, you're at work, right? And you're doing whatever it is that your job entails. Then at five-ish, to help you decompress, it's probably not a bad time, if it's not stressful, to call a family member or something like that.

PEGGY: What's going on in our circadian rhythm? What's happening hormonally, or...?

DR BREUS: Sure. When we look at the hormones and the circadian rhythms at this point – and, again, we're talking primarily about seniors for this discussion – what's happening is you're going towards the tail end of the day. You're probably going to be having dinner around five-thirty, six. Then you're going to be moving into the rest of your evening. So what do we want to do with the rest of our evening?

As we said before, there are a lot of people who have a tendency to just go to bed because they don't have anything left to do. They're just kind of wrapping up – their day is done and they want to be able to wake up at five, so they figure they should go to bed at nine. And that might be okay as long as that rhythm is working for you.

PEGGY: If it's consistent.

DR BREUS: If it's consistent, and it's working for you. But let's say that you have a cocktail, and you're hanging out for dinner, have a glass of wine, or a beer, or what have you... then is that a bad time at that point to relax?

It's not a bad time to relax, but if you've decided to drink alcohol, be careful. Number one, depending upon what time you take your medication, it can interact with your medications.

But, number two, alcohol can depress you. It can depress all of your senses, and it can make you feel sleepy earlier than you probably want to. So limit it to one glass of wine or one beer. You probably don't want to go more than that, because otherwise what ends up happening is that, depending on what time you drink alcohol, it can have a different effect. There's a reason it's called "happy hour."

PEGGY: Aha!

DR BREUS: Right? So when you drink alcohol at a particular time in your circadian rhythm it's uplifting. When you drink it later on in the evening, it's depressing.

PEGGY: It's a nightcap.

DR BREUS: Exactly.

PEGGY: We don't want the nightcap.

DR BREUS: You know, it's interesting when you look at data on nightcaps. If people have a hard time falling asleep, should they have one glass of something, and will it affect them?

It's probably not the worst idea I've heard, but at the end of the day there's a big difference between alcohol-filled sleep and natural sleep. So I tell people, if you're going to have one drink before you go to bed, give yourself a good hour for your body to digest it.

PEGGY: Okay. So now we're having a nice, healthy dinner...

DR BREUS: Right.

PEGGY: But not a huge meal.

DR BREUS: Not at all.

PEGGY: Because we don't want to overeat when we're sleeping.

DR BREUS: Yes, and people say that lunch should be the biggest meal of the day, or breakfast should be the biggest meal of the day. What I would tell you is, the biggest thing you need to think about is the *size* of your dinner.

A lot of people don't eat much for breakfast, don't eat much for lunch, and then they have this really big dinner, and it's just like a rock in their stomach. It takes the body a lot to metabolize through that.

What you really want to do is you want to have a lunch-sized dinner, and a dinner-sized lunch.

PEGGY: Switch.

DR BREUS: Exactly.

PEGGY: To work with your circadian rhythm.

DR BREUS: Yeah.

PEGGY: Because then your body doesn't have so much work to do at night to digest this heavy load in there.

DR BREUS: Right. Absolutely.

PEGGY: Okay.

DR BREUS: So you get it!

PEGGY: I get it. So we're past dinnertime. Now we've got evening, and what would be good? Social activities? Playing cards with friends?

DR BREUS: Absolutely. Playing cards with friends, going to the movies, talking on the telephone. Watching TV isn't a horrible activity. It only gets bad if that's all you do, right? If you're watching television for four or five hours in an evening, that's probably not the best idea for you.

PEGGY: Right.

DR BREUS: I like especially for my senior patients to do something that's got a little bit of an intellectual side to it. Whether it's Sudoku, or a crossword, or find-the-word puzzles, or having a conversation, playing cards, playing a game...

Whatever it is, just make it something to keep a little bit more mental stimulation going. I like that idea for people in the later afternoon – or evening, rather – because, number one, it helps give you something to do, as opposed to falling asleep. It's stimulating, but not so stimulating that it's going to keep you awake.

Like, you don't want to play poker for a lot of money late at night, because then you're worried about the money! But if you're hanging out with your friends playing bridge, there's nothing wrong with that.

PEGGY: That's really good. Speaking of hanging out with friends, we know that that's absolutely one of the best things you can do for your brain – to have social interactions, to not isolate yourself, and to be involved with other people.

DR BREUS: Right.

PEGGY: So this might be a good time to do these activities.

DR BREUS: There's no question. I think it's a perfect time to do those activities. Number one, it takes up that space of time, and then sometimes you can have dinner during those activities, right?

So good activities are going out with friends for a meal, and then going to a movie... or going and playing cards at somebody's house where they're serving food, or something like that. You just have to be a little bit careful and remember the amount of food that you're going to bring on.

PEGGY: And the amount of alcohol.

DR BREUS: And the amount of alcohol.

PEGGY: So now we're getting ready for bed. You know, speaking of getting ready for bed, let's discuss the issues. Because many people are on their computers, or phones, or tablets, and they may not realize that what they're doing is affecting their circadian rhythms.

DR BREUS: So it is. We now know that that blue light that's emitted either from the television, your laptop, your mobile device, like a phone or a tablet – actually can have an effect. But I'm the only sleep doctor in the universe who says it's okay to fall asleep with the TV on.

PEGGY: Aha!

DR BREUS: And I'll tell you why, okay? Because I have some patients who say they can't turn off their brain at night. And if they watch television, what they do is they don't really watch it. It's on, their eyes are closed, and they're just listening to the television, and it's enough of a distraction from whatever might be stressing them out or bothering them to allow them to then coast off into sleep.

95% of the televisions that are made today have a timer built into the software. If you can figure out how to work it –

PEGGY: That's a tall order.

DR BREUS: Right! Or get your son, or your daughter, or your grandchild or whoever to teach you how to use it. You might be surprised at how easy it is to turn the TV off.

What I don't like, though, is when people have a tablet late at night, or a phone.

PEGGY: Or they're on the computer.

DR BREUS: Yes, because the proximity of the light is much closer to your face than a television. You know, your television's all the way across the room. And then the level of engagement is different, too.

If I'm watching "Seinfeld" to help me fall asleep, I'm really not paying a whole lot of attention. But if I'm reading an email from a close friend or I'm playing a game and trying to get my high score or something like that, the level of engagement can have a pretty big effect.

I like to do what I call an "electronic curfew." Approximately one hour, hour-and-a-half before bed, electronics go off – other than television, if that's what you want to do.

PEGGY: Right.

DR BREUS: I'd plug your phone in someplace different, put your computer down. You don't have to check your last email. There's no emergency that's going on.

PEGGY: Probably not.

DR BREUS: Well, if it is, it's certainly not coming to you in an email. Give yourself some time to chill out.

The big thing that people forget is that sleep is not an on/off switch. It's more like slowly pulling your foot off the gas, and slowly putting your foot on the brake.

PEGGY: Getting yourself in the mood and the proper mental place to achieve it.

DR BREUS: Yes, it's like that. Exactly. So I came up with a technique for people that I call "The Power-Down Hour."

PEGGY: Take us through your Power-Down Hour.

DR BREUS: Let's say that your bedtime is ten o'clock, okay? Then nine is when electronics are gone. You're going to set your electronics curfew. And then, starting at nine you're going to break that last hour before bed into three distinct parts.

The first 20 minutes are just things you've got to do before the next day. So in our house we're getting backpacks together for the kids. I might be getting my briefcase out and getting ready for the next day. 20 minutes – got to do it in 20 minutes, or it's done.

20 minutes for hygiene – brush your teeth, wash your face – whatever it is. By the way, one of the interesting things that a lot of people forget is if they have really bright lights in their bathroom, and then they go in there at night to remove makeup, or brush their teeth, or things like that, it can actually prevent them from being able to fall asleep. Install a dimmer switch in your bathroom and have dim light while you're doing that. You'll actually fall asleep a lot easier.

PEGGY: Ooh.

DR BREUS: The third thing you want to do is some form of meditation or relaxation for about 20 minutes. You want to do it in bed, preferably with the light off. And that can be anything from deep breathing, like what we've been talking about, meditation, prayer.

If you want to read, read Scripture or a good fiction book. Steer clear of non-fiction books at night. They have a tendency to make you think too much.

PEGGY: Well, how about mysteries? Because you don't want to keep reading to have to stay up to find out who did it.

DR BREUS: Well, see, what I like about fiction – and mysteries in particular – is when the chapter's done, the chapter's done, and you can put your book down and pick it up later. So I think it's okay to read those kinds of things. Maybe not a murder mystery, or a horror story, or something along those lines.

PEGGY: Right.

DR BREUS: Then once you've finished that, you really should be allowing your body to coast right into sleep.

PEGGY: Okay. So now we've set up kind of a "sleep hygiene program"...

DR BREUS: Correct.

PEGGY: ...where we have a regular routine, and our body... what's going on inside our body when we do that? I mean, are hormones changing? What is going on internally to make that work for us?

DR BREUS: There are a lot of different hormones in your body that do a lot of different things, but let's talk about two big ones that people have probably heard about that affect sleep.

One is something called "cortisol" and the other is called "melatonin."

So, cortisol is the stress hormone. The more stressed you are, the more cortisol you have, right? And the thing is, is you don't want high levels of cortisol at night, because –

PEGGY: You can't sleep.

DR BREUS: You can't sleep. That's right. And not only are you stressed, but cortisol will linger. It's hard to get cortisol out of your system once a certain level of it has kind of gotten in there—right? – from stress.

So let's say you're driving home and you get this horrible phone call about some tragedy that's occurred. There goes your cortisol. You're not going to sleep because you can't turn your brain off, because your cortisol level is so high... yadda, yadda, yadda. It makes it much more difficult to fall asleep.

But, the second hormone is melatonin, and that's the one you do want to be high at night. You actually want the opposite to occur in the morning. You want high levels of cortisol in the morning to wake you up and get you going, and low levels of melatonin.

They actually work in what's called a "phase response curve." What we see in the morning is a high level of cortisol, and then throughout the day we see it slowly dipping, dipping, dipping, dipping, dipping... and then getting low right before bed.

The opposite is true of melatonin. In the morning it's at its lowest, and then slowly it increases throughout the day and gets high towards the end. And that's really hormonally what we're looking at.

PEGGY: What you're describing is if we set our bodies by maintaining these regular schedules and doing things at their optimal time...

DR BREUS: Right. Exactly.

PEGGY: ...we're going to make the melatonin when we need it, and make the cortisol when we need it, too.

DR BREUS: Right.

PEGGY: And we're not going to take melatonin. And tell us – melatonin may be the most popular sleep supplement?

DR BREUS: It is. It's the most popular sleep supplement. And there are things to think about when you're talking about melatonin.

First of all, what's the correct dose? The correct dose is between a half and one milligram. So the 3 mg, 5 mg, 10 mg doses that you see out there in many supplements are all in overdosage format.

PEGGY: I don't think I've ever seen one that low. Or maybe they're there, but you have to look for them.

DR BREUS: They are. You've got to look for them. I found them online, and I actually found them at Trader Joe's, of all places.

PEGGY: Oh, okay, there you go.

DR BREUS: So if you've got one of those nearby, you might be able to get one.

PEGGY: Okay.

DR BREUS: Number two is, you should take melatonin 90 minutes before bed. It takes that long for plasma [blood] concentration levels to reach that level, especially when we talk about seniors who are slower metabolizers. It takes a while for the melatonin in the supplement to get where you want it to go.

Melatonin is not a sleeping pill. It's not a sleep initiator. It's a circadian rhythm regulator. There's a big difference there. But I don't necessarily have a big problem with people taking melatonin as they get into their senior years, because once you hit about 55, 65, you actually start producing less melatonin.

Now don't get me wrong. I am not telling everybody who is in that age range to run out and start putting themselves on melatonin. But what I am saying is if you find that you're having significant difficulty falling asleep – but primarily, staying asleep – melatonin could be a supplement that might be worthwhile for you.

Be sure to check with your doctor because melatonin can interact with certain medications, specifically high blood pressure medications.

PEGGY: Well, I'm glad you raised the topic of medications, because we're talking about seniors.

DR BREUS: Sure.

PEGGY: And many of them are on many medications, which may be interacting with each other. Are some of these affecting their quality of sleep?

DR BREUS: No question about it. And we should also talk about sleeping pills, right?

PEGGY: Let's talk about sleeping pills.

DR BREUS: Right. There are lots of medications out there, and if you read the labels, almost all of them either make you tired or make you unable to sleep, right?

PEGGY: Not good.

DR BREUS: Not good in either direction, so I'm a big "less medicine is better" kind of person. I'm not saying don't take medicine. I'm not saying be afraid of medicine. Medicine can be extremely helpful, but just speak with your doctor about getting the lowest effective dose.

Sleeping pills are a whole different ballgame. There's a lot, a lot, a lot of people out there who are taking sleeping pills, and there are all kinds.

PEGGY: We're talking about prescription sleeping pills.

DR BREUS: We are. Well, we can talk about either. We can talk about prescription sleeping pills, or we can talk about over-the-counter sleeping aids.

PEGGY: Let's begin with the prescription ones, because millions of people are on them.

DR BREUS: They are. Other than thyroid medication, it's actually one of the most heavily prescribed classes of medication out there.

It turns out there are three different classes of sleep medication. There's what are called the "non-benzodiazepine hypnotics" – Ambien, Lunesta, those types of medications.

PEGGY: Okay.

DR BREUS: There are the benzodiazepines, which were originally anxiety medications, like Valium, or Xanax, or Restoril. There's another class of sleeping pills which are actually anti-depressants – Trazodone is a big one. Celexa is one that can actually be quite helpful for sleep.

The question becomes, do you really need a sleeping pill?

I'm of the belief that some people out there may have a "broken sleeper," right, that switch in their head that makes them fall asleep. But most people don't have "a broken sleeper." Very few people have that where it's broken.

PEGGY: Right.

DR BREUS: But what's happened is they've had a bad situation – death of a loved one, a health scare – something that's caused a high level of stress, which elevates cortisol, which makes it hard to sleep.

So what do they do? That stress isn't necessarily going away. It happens for three days, five days, ten days... And then they talk to their doctor and say something like, "Doc, I'm really not sleeping."

So the doctor gives them a pill. That pill decreases the stress, makes them fall asleep, and then they associate falling asleep with the pill.

PEGGY: It becomes a psychological dependence?

DR BREUS: Exactly. And with so many of the sleep aids – the Ambiens and Lunestas of the world – there's very little data to suggest that they are physiologically addictive. Nobody's out there "jonesing" for an Ambien, right? It doesn't have any street value. But psychologically speaking, it's one of the most difficult drugs to get away from a patient.

PEGGY: That's scary, because taking drugs like Ambien is also associated with driving accidents, with increased falls, and as you know, for seniors that means winding up in the emergency room.

DR BREUS: Correct. Right. It's really interesting, too, that when you look at the data very, very closely, it turns out that a lot of people actually mix alcohol with the sleep aid.

PEGGY: Ooh, that's bad.

DR BREUS: What they'll do is they'll have a glass or two of wine with dinner, and then it might be three or four hours later, and they're no longer feeling the effects of alcohol, and then they take their nightly sleeping pill. That's when the problems occur, more so than not.

PEGGY: You made a really interesting point. It's a very helpful way to think about the idea that there's not a sleep switch that's broken. In other words, you could have a heart problem because over time your heart is wearing out, and there are physical problems in the heart.

But you're saying when you're having problems with sleep, there isn't a physical malfunction going on. It's just that you're not optimizing your body's natural rhythm.

DR BREUS: You're doing two things: You're not optimizing your body's natural rhythm, you've got that 100% correct, and that's what my whole book *The Power of When* is about...

PEGGY: *The Power of When,* right.

DR BREUS: But also, the other thing is, there's a mental aspect to sleep. 75% of the reasons why people either don't fall asleep or stay asleep involve either anxiety or depression.

PEGGY: Okay.

DR BREUS: Right? So what's going on in your world that's bothering you? That can have a dramatic effect on your sleep.

One of the techniques I use with a lot of my patients is something called a "worry journal." Remember that Power-Down Hour I was talking about before?

PEGGY: Yes, yes.

DR BREUS: Well then, right before the Power-Down Hour starts, if you've got some things on your mind, write them down. Just take a piece of paper, draw a line down the middle. Put every problem that you have on one side, and then one solution on the other.

Now, you don't have to solve the problem. The solution might be, "I'm going to think about this problem tomorrow at ten AM when I'm sharp."

PEGGY: Like Scarlett O'Hara – "I'll think about it tomorrow."

DR BREUS: Right. Tomorrow is another day, right? So you want to think about doing it that way, because thinking right before sleep elevates cortisol, elevates autonomic arousal and makes it difficult to sleep. When you go to sleep, you really want to be kind of coasting in to the evening, and not be full of thought.

Now, it's easy to say; it's not always so easy to do. But a worry journal's a great way for people to reduce stress. And it also helps them plan their next day. "Oh, you know what? I was thinking about this yesterday. I need to call so-and-so's teacher. I need to call my granddaughter, and to do whatever I need to do. I've got that scheduled. I don't have to worry about it anymore."

PEGGY: I wrote it down.

DR BREUS: Right.

PEGGY: I don't have to worry about remembering it.

DR BREUS: Exactly.

PEGGY: Also, when you're talking about depression and anxiety preventing sleep... the way you've taken us through the day, we've done things that have helped us with that. We've been outside. We've had exposure to vitamin D.

DR BREUS: To sunlight, yup. Big deal.

PEGGY: And we've gotten some exercise.

DR BREUS: And some breathing.

PEGGY: Some breathing. These are all things that – studies have shown – can ameliorate depression and anxiety.

DR BREUS: Absolutely. Natural anxiety and depression reducers – all the things I'm talking about.

PEGGY: That's one reason people may not sleep well – because of these kinds of stresses in their life.

DR BREUS: Sure. Right.

PEGGY: And then there are the physical aspects of getting older, where you might be snoring and have sleep apnea and some of those kinds of issues, so...

DR BREUS: And there's another one that we haven't even discussed – pain.

PEGGY: Pain, pain.

DR BREUS: Right, pain is a big factor when it comes to sleep, because you might have low back pain. You might have chronic fatigue. You might have some medical ailment that's giving you pain in the middle of the night...

PEGGY: Arthritis.

DR BREUS: Arthritis is another big one, right. For some people, the only time they can actually find relief from their pain is when they lie down, right, because they're up and around during the day, and they've got joint issues or what have you.

Some people, if they move wrong in their sleep, it wakes them up, and then they're up for the night, and that can be an issue as well.

PEGGY: So what are we going to do for those people?

DR BREUS: It's kind of interesting. I actually find that with some of those people, some of the PM's, like Advil PM, the nighttime analgesics, can work quite well. Again, talk with your doctor. Make sure it doesn't interact with anything. Make sure they're okay with it.

But for example, I work in a pain center one day a month because people in pain don't sleep. So I've studied this relationship, and here's what I've learned: You have to treat them both. You have to treat the pain and the sleeplessness at the same time. You can't just treat the pain and hope that the sleep gets better, or give the patient a sleeping pill and hope that the pain gets better.

PEGGY: Right. No.

DR BREUS: It doesn't seem to work. You have to treat them both at the same time. And some of these over-the-counter alternatives can actually be quite helpful. The problem comes in if you take them every night for months and months and months at a time.

PEGGY: Yes, then they start having other effects.

DR BREUS: Well, they actually stop working, and then people have to take more, thinking it's going to work better, and then before you know it you're taking five, eight, ten of these a night.

PEGGY: This is not good.

DR BREUS: That's not good.

PEGGY: This is not good. Now also, talking about pain, if you're in pain and you can't sleep, it seems that that would bring on anxiety and depression so that they would create a kind of cycle, which isn't good.

DR BREUS: Exactly. It's a cycle, absolutely.

PEGGY: So we've got pain, and have we talked about snoring, sleep apnea? I mean, these are physical problems. And then people get up and go to the bathroom at night. So those are other things that...

DR BREUS: Absolutely.

PEGGY: How do we address all that? Let's begin with sleep apnea – so many older people probably develop it, among other things, and it's correlated with weight gain.

DR BREUS: Sure. They do. We know that as we get older our musculature is not as taut as it once was. We're not in as good a shape, right? It's unfortunate, but that's just how it is, right?

PEGGY: That's the human body.

DR BREUS: Right, and one of the big things we see is that the throat begins to get more and more narrow and closed. And we gain weight, which puts pressure on this, so when we lie down, that adipose [fat] tissue can push against that already narrow throat. And that's when we see sleep apnea.

It's kind of interesting when you look at men versus women for sleep apnea. There are usually two men for every one woman. But as soon as a woman hits menopause, it's even.

PEGGY: Oh. And what happens to the woman?

DR BREUS: She gains weight, and her hormones change, and it actually can cause a slight narrowing of the throat, and then that added weight. It's tough, but if you can keep your weight down you will be in much better shape from a physical standpoint, but also from a sleep standpoint.

But sleep apnea can really have some pretty major effects. And remember, sleep apnea is when you stop breathing at night and your throat actually collapses. So then you either have to use a breathing machine called a "CPAP machine," which helps open up that airway. Or there are now mouthpieces that people can use that have got an upper and a lower to bring your jaw forward, open it up. There are also surgeries, but I'm not a big fan of surgery.

PEGGY: Yeah, they're difficult.

DR BREUS: They're very hard to recover from.

PEGGY: Yeah, they're complicated. So we've now gone through our whole day. We've gotten up in the morning at the same time, and we've hydrated. First thing, we have some water.

DR BREUS: Yup.

PEGGY: And we've walked outside. We've had sun. Now we're going to sleep at night. What's our rhythm looking like at night? Take us through that successful night of sleep. What is the rhythm?

DR BREUS: Sure. We've turned off our electronics an hour before bed. We're in the midst of our Power-Down Hour, right? 20 minutes of stuff you've just got to do, 20 minutes of hygiene, and we're now in the final phase of that 20 minutes of some form of relaxation.

So that's where I think we get all of the good stuff going on, to allow us to coast into sleep in an easier way.

Some people do different things. I personally recommend for people the deep breathing, or the relaxation. There are some wonderful tapes out there that you can get that do guided imagery, muscle relaxation – things like that. And when you start to look at people's hormones, when they participate in those activities, everything starts to go down. Melatonin starts to rise, and that's what we're looking for.

PEGGY: In a natural way. And then, do we need our REM sleep? What's going to happen, actually, during the night?

DR BREUS: Mother Nature's going to take care of all of that for us, which is great.

PEGGY: Okay.

DR BREUS: The only thing that we know is that, as seniors, the amplitude or the height of the brainwaves begins to shrink. It's just that the brain isn't firing off the brainwaves that it used to when we were 13, or 18, or 20, or what have you. You're still getting decent quality sleep, but you definitely need to follow these rules a little bit more strictly the older you get because it's tough, and there's a lot of other factors.

The biggest other factor for my senior patients is medication. If they're on a medication for some type of ailment, we know there are significant side effects from those.

PEGGY: And that's going to affect the waves of the sleep levels they reach?

DR BREUS: They are.

PEGGY: So they may not get into that deepest level of sleep...?

DR BREUS: It depends on how you look at it. I would say the deepest level of sleep is Stages 3 and 4, because the brain is the least active during that stage. But believe it or not, during REM sleep, the sleep where your eyes move back and forth when you dream, would you believe me if I told you that your brain is almost as active as when you're awake?

PEGGY: Yeah, I would, because...

DR BREUS: You're dreaming, right? You've got all kinds of stuff going on.

PEGGY: Yeah. It looks active.

DR BREUS: Right. It is. It's very active.

So I'll mention a couple of quick tricks that I teach my seniors who are having problems when they're falling asleep. Number one, if your mind is just going, going, going, this is going to sound silly, but it really works: Count backwards from 300 by 3's.

PEGGY: Whoa! That's hard work!

DR BREUS: It's mathematically so complicated you can't think of anything else, and it's so doggone boring, you're out like a light.

PEGGY: Huh.

DR BREUS: Works like a charm.

PEGGY: Good.

DR BREUS: My famous recipe for banana tea.

PEGGY: Banana tea – tell us about banana tea.

DR BREUS: Magnesium turns out to be really sleep-inducing – calming the muscles, calming everything down. There's a tremendous amount of magnesium in bananas, but there's three times the amount of magnesium in the peel, rather than the fruit.

So what I have my patients do is wash off the banana – get any dirt or pesticides off. Cut off the tips, cut it in half. Leave the peel on and the fruit in it. Put it in about three or four cups of boiling water and let it boil for about four or five minutes, and then take the water and put that into your teacup and drink the water. If you like bananas, it's delicious, and it's got so much magnesium it'll put you out like a light.

PEGGY: And so we have that cup of tea at night.

DR BREUS: Yeah. You can have it, for example, right before that 20 minutes of meditation and relaxation.

PEGGY: Oh, how lovely – a cup of banana tea.

DR BREUS: Exactly. Works out well.

PEGGY: And then count down from 300. I'm very busy.

DR BREUS: 300. You'll be done.

PEGGY: With my drinking, and my counting, very busy. And any other tips?

DR BREUS: Light is a big one. When you look at the light that's in your bedroom, it's great to install dimmer switches, or keep that light at a lower level. Because remember, light stops the production of melatonin, and melatonin is our friend in the evening. It's one of the things that helps us sleep.

So you don't want to have your bedroom really well lit. You want to be able to have a dimmer sort of atmosphere. If you like to read before bed, use a book light, as opposed to a bedside table light.

PEGGY: Alright.

DR BREUS: A book light will focus the light exactly where it needs to be. It's not in your eyes, whereas if you have a bedside table lamp, it can have an effect.

PEGGY: Excellent. So we're reading a book – a fiction book, not a non-fiction book.

DR BREUS: Fiction book, not non-fiction.

PEGGY: We're drinking our banana tea.

DR BREUS: Yeah.

PEGGY: And then we're meditating and counting backwards from 300, and we're gone.

DR BREUS: Yup.

PEGGY: Seven-and-one-half hours later, we wake up, we feel great.

DR BREUS: Exactly. It's that simple.

PEGGY: And we say, "Thank you, Dr. Breus."

DR BREUS: It is that simple, I promise.

PEGGY: Well, thank you so much for coming today and telling us how we can use natural rhythms in our body to protect our brain, basically, for the long haul.

DR BREUS: You know, it's great to be able to talk about this type of science with everybody, and the techniques should be ones that are so easy for people to do. If people want to learn more about my book or what I'm doing, they can come to www.thepowerofwhen.com.

PEGGY: www.thepowerofwhen.com. Well, thank you so much for coming, Dr. Breus, and thank you for watching. I hope you learned a lot of valuable information about how you can work with your body's natural rhythms to optimize your mental energy and protect your brain.

Interview with Mary Kay Ross, M.D., F.A.C.E.P.

PEGGY SARLIN: Hello. I'm Peggy Sarlin, and today I'm in New York with Dr. Mary Kay Ross, who's going to tell us about the great results she's getting with patients with Alzheimer's by using the Bredesen Protocol.

And specifically, we're going to talk today about environmental toxins, common ones like mold, and how they can affect your brain.

Dr. Ross is the owner and the founder of the Institute for Personalized Medicine in Savannah, Georgia, and she's one of just a few hundred doctors who's actually trained with Dr. Dale Bredesen in this protocol for treating Alzheimer's.

So welcome, Dr. Ross.

DR MARY KAY ROSS: Thank you, Peggy. Thank you for having me.

PEGGY: Well, it's a pleasure to have you here. I want to begin by asking you about your own personal story. You were an emergency room physician, and now you've made a big change, and you practice functional medicine. So what precipitated that change?

DR ROSS: Well, I actually became a patient. I was exposed to mold in my home and became very ill. I developed respiratory problems, I developed thyroid problems, and I developed autoimmune disease. I had psoriatic arthritis, and in an effort to heal myself and find out, really, what my ailments were coming from and what I could do about them, I became involved in functional medicine.

I trained at the Institute for Functional Medicine, and it's become a big passion of mine. I've discovered, really, what a poor job traditional medicine does for chronic illness.

PEGGY: For chronic illness, that's an important point. Functional medicine is particularly suited to treating people with chronic illnesses.

DR ROSS: That's correct. That's right.

PEGGY: Okay. So let's go back. This whole life change for you was a kind of random thing that happened to you because of exposure to mold. So tell us about that. What happens to people who are exposed to mold? What happens to their brains?

DR ROSS: It can have a very bad effect on your brain, obviously, and it can be a cause for Alzheimer's disease. Dr. Bredesen actually wrote a paper on inhalational Alzheimer's disease.

Mold is a biotoxin, and we now know that 25% of the population have a genetic predisposition to mold susceptibility, or biotoxin susceptibility. And 25% is a pretty large group of people. Their immune system really doesn't pick up on the toxins that they're being exposed to. So it damages their immune system.

Mold, in particular, through breathing in the spores and the mycotoxins, can actually cause a great deal of inflammation, and can cause Alzheimer's disease in certain patients.

PEGGY: Dr. Ross, you used a phrase that I think most people have never heard – that's "inhalation Alzheimer's". That's a new thought for people, I think. It means that you have activated Alzheimer's in your brain by breathing in something through your nose. Is that right?

DR ROSS: That's absolutely correct.

PEGGY: And what you've breathed in is something in your home.

DR ROSS: It's kind of a crazy notion. We all live in buildings. We all live in homes, and we think of that as our safe haven. But in reality, we build our buildings out of mold food. We all have plumbing inside our walls that runs water, and we all have the capability of having leaks. It takes 30 to 36 hours to grow mold.

PEGGY: Wow!

DR ROSS: And oftentimes, you're never aware of it.

PEGGY: So the mold is always related to water damage, in every case?

DR ROSS: It's always related to either humidity or water. It's always going to be a wet/damp environment.

PEGGY: Does that mean that people who live in humid parts of the country might not have had a plumbing problem, but it's just humid, and so there's mold? Is that happening a lot?

DR ROSS: It can be. For example, I live in Savannah. If you don't have your HVAC properly done, and I certainly can't explain that to you, but the humidity...

PEGGY: That's okay.

DR ROSS: ...can cause mold to grow in the HVAC system. And then, of course, when you turn it on, you'll be spreading it throughout the house.

PEGGY: So you're spreading it through the house. You're inhaling it, and you may be actually causing inhalation Alzheimer's.

DR ROSS: Absolutely.

PEGGY: How many doctors know about inhalational Alzheimer's? What are your chances of going to your local physician, neurologist, whatever, and having them say, "That's inhalational Alzheimer's".

DR ROSS: Probably not very many.

PEGGY: How do you know that's what it is? Tell us about some patients for whom this is the problem, and what you've done for them.

DR ROSS: I have been trained, obviously, by Dr. Bredesen. So when I approach a patient, I'm looking for the big picture. I'm looking for everything. I want to know more about their environment and their exposures.

So when they have a history of a leak in their house, which oftentimes they do, we look for the inflammatory markers, and those will usually be elevated. We do mycotoxin testing in their urine so we can determine that they've been exposed to mycotoxins, which are created by toxic molds. And then we test their house, and we look at the mold that we find in the house.

PEGGY: In the house.

DR ROSS: Then we can take that test and compare it to the mycotoxins. And really, you can correlate the exposure to what you're seeing in the patient.

PEGGY: Okay, so you test the patient, and you see very specifically that it looks like they've been exposed to this particular kind of toxin. What's a mycotoxin?

DR ROSS: A mycotoxin is created by a toxic mold, so it's the toxin that the mold creates. It's something that isn't metabolically active, so you really can't kill it, and it's something that's a very, very small particle. So it can stay in the furniture. You can breathe it in.

It can cause inflammation in your body. Once it gets in there, then it increases the inflammation and the chemicals that are released in your body, the cytokines, and it can cause the damage.

We now believe that in Alzheimer's, for example, the plaques we have in our brain, or that are in the brains of the Alzheimer's patients, develop because our bodies actually make those plaques in an effort to help you.

PEGGY: That's a very important point, and I think we should look at that for a moment, because there have been so many disappointing tests for medications for Alzheimer's.

You know, every week you see some other disaster, a failed trial for something that was going to be the great new drug. And most of them seem to be aiming to remove the plaque. "Oh, people with Alzheimer's have this plaque; let's take away the plaque."

You're saying – and Dr. Bredesen is saying – that plaque is protective, that it's some kind of a shield that the brain is expressing to protect itself from these toxins, from the mold.

DR ROSS: I think it's an effort on the body's part to protect you. Certainly, we think the plaques are a problem, and we can remove them, or try to remove them. But you also want to understand why they're there, and you want to remove the insult that caused your body to make the plaque.

PEGGY: So the insult, the insult of the exposure to mold, which was on your furniture, it's in your rug, it's in your walls... Where is it? It's...

DR ROSS: It can be in so many places.

PEGGY: And some people are more genetically predisposed than others to react to these toxins. So you can have, for example, a husband and a wife, and they're living in the same house, and one person is getting very sick from it, and the other one's somehow managing. What's going on in their bodies?

DR ROSS: That's correct. Depending on their genetics, there is a big difference in the response that people have to their exposure.

For example, the couple that I have as patients, they were my first Bredesen patients. She actually has the Alzheimer's, but he, on the other hand, has all kinds of respiratory problems. He actually had a collapsed lung that we believe may be related. He also has had some cognitive issues, but nothing on the scope that she's had.

PEGGY: That's actually fascinating. So they have the same exposure to mold, but in her, it precipitates Alzheimer's – inhalational Alzheimer's, a new term that we're learning now – and he has respiratory problems. He's got a whole other thing going on. But it's the same cause, and a doctor would not necessarily make that relationship. "Oh, you're both suffering from mold."

DR ROSS: That's right.

PEGGY: So you need a very sophisticated medical detective to figure out what they have in common. So how do you help these people?

DR ROSS: We've managed to try and get them out of their exposure. That's the first thing that you need to do. We used binders to remove the mycotoxins.

PEGGY: Tell us what a binder is.

DR ROSS: There are many different types of binders, but the one I typically use is prescription, and it's cholestyramine.

So cholestyramine is an older drug. It's been used for a very long time for cholesterol, but it does help with toxins, and it removes them through the hepatobiliary system. It actually binds bile, and it's an easy drug to use, and it's not expensive. You can get it from any pharmacy, and it really helps, and it helps people regain clarity when they remove the toxins.

PEGGY: So the term "binder," which we may not be familiar with, means something that's going to attach itself to something you don't want, to the toxin.

DR ROSS: That's correct.

PEGGY: It's going to bind to it, and then it's going to escort it out of your body.

DR ROSS: That's right. That's absolutely right.

PEGGY: Okay. And would most doctors know that they can prescribe this drug?

DR ROSS: You know, I don't think that most doctors are aware of that. I certainly wasn't until I had trained at IFM. And there, you were only given a little preliminary bit of information, and then the rest of it I obtained from Dr. Shoemaker.

PEGGY: Okay, tell us about Dr. Shoemaker. He's done a lot of work in this area.

DR ROSS: Dr. Ritchie Shoemaker is a biotoxin physician, and he has basically discovered biotoxins, and he has been treating them. He's come up with a protocol, and he trains many other physicians who follow this protocol.

So Dr. Shoemaker uses cholestyramine to remove the toxins. He does have some other things, other medications that he uses, that sometimes we use, and sometimes we don't. Predominantly, what I do is use functional medicine. So supporting the diet, supporting the exercise, supporting the person using mindfulness training. I use quite a few nutraceuticals, and then I use cholestyramine as well.

Again, I have to emphasize, it's so important to get out of the house, out of the exposure, or they're not going to get better.

PEGGY: Tell us about some patients that you successfully treated. And I know people are going to want to hear, if you'd talk about nutraceuticals, if you talk about supplements that you've given them. They're going to want to know what they are, and, you know, even brand names...

DR ROSS: Absolutely. First of all, I'll tell you a happy story. Let me give you a little bit of an idea of what happens at the end of the day, and what people can expect, and what kind of an outcome they can look forward to. Because it's a pretty bleak picture up until now, and actually, people are getting better.

I'm finding I have many, many patients that actually are starting to be able to take care of their own protocol. There's somebody who couldn't drive, and now they're driving. Many patients who are mothers of teenagers who now get in the car and drive with their teenagers. They're cooking dinner. They're able to follow recipes.

PEGGY: This is great.

DR ROSS: They go to the grocery... they're starting to get their lives back, and they're able to function, and I think that that's really the goal that we all have.

PEGGY: To be able to drive... to be able to cook...to just be able to live, to handle the tasks of daily life. These people have been so affected. Their cognitive powers have been so diminished that they couldn't even do the routines of daily life.

DR ROSS: That's right.

PEGGY: Wow, that's serious stuff. Okay, so what are the happy outcomes? Tell us about some of your patients.

DR ROSS: Okay, I have a patient that's 52 years old, and she moved into a very old home. She was very healthy, a very well-educated engineer, and had a family with teenagers and college students. And suddenly, she developed Alzheimer's.

Her family really didn't see it coming initially, and then when they realized it, it was full-blown Alzheimer's. She had had an amyloid scan that was positive.

We did a lot of history taking, and realized that she had had a lot of leaks in the house. It was very old. We tested the house, and the mold was through the roof in the house.

So she had to move out of the house. But she's actually getting better now. She's starting to drive with her children. She's actually going to the grocery with family members, actively shopping, putting her protocol together...

In the beginning, she couldn't do any of that. She's doing her brain studies every day. She works on brain exercises, and we're seeing great movement in the right direction.

PEGGY: One thing that occurred to me when you were describing this young woman, this 52-year-old woman who's suddenly stricken with Alzheimer's...is this perhaps a clue that the timeline of developing the Alzheimer's can be short – in other words, that it comes on much more quickly? It's not the gradual decline that we see.

So if somebody suddenly goes downhill, might that be clue that there's a toxic exposure?

DR ROSS: Absolutely. And in a lot of these people, it seems – and I mentioned this earlier – to be related to hormones as well. So it's sort of that perfect storm that happens in their lives.

Here you have a vibrant person who's in their 50s. They're active. They're busy. They're well-educated. And suddenly, they're going through menopause, and they have stress on their body – and the stress can actually be the stress of a house that's not healthy – and especially if they have the HLA predisposition to being ill by mold.

PEGGY: So you have somebody who's going through a hormonal change of life. They may have a genetic predisposition to be more affected by toxins like mold.

DR ROSS: That's correct.

PEGGY: And then they're exposed to mold, plus who knows? There may be other factors – they might not be eating in the healthiest manner, and all those other things.

So you treated this woman who came to you, a previously healthy woman who was living in a house with mold. Tell us specifically some of the nutraceuticals.

DR ROSS: We did the high-fat diet, and we use MCT oil, and I particularly like Brain Octane Oil.

PEGGY: Brain Octane Oil is a brand? Is that what we're talking about?

DR ROSS: It's a brand. It's made by Bulletproof, and it's actually something that when you start taking it, you have to start at a very low dose, one teaspoon, and build up slowly, because it can cause some adverse G.I. effects. But other than that, it's something that I really see a lot of benefit with.

So she's on the Brain Octane Oil. We make sure that we've done some genetic testing. So if she has, for instance, MTHFR, we fix that.

PEGGY: That's the genetic predisposition.

DR ROSS: That's a genetic problem that you can have that will not give you the predisposition to mold, but it makes it so your body doesn't detox well.

PEGGY: Oh.

DR ROSS: So if you also have that against you, you don't methylate well. Methylation is a chemical reaction in our body, and people that don't methylate well don't detox well.

And if your detox pathways aren't working well, and you have the genetic predisposition, it makes it very hard for your body to deal with these toxins. There are supplements that we use for that as well. I use a lot of Orthomolecular brand.

PEGGY: This is over-the-counter?

DR ROSS: People would have to get it through a physician.

PEGGY: Oh.

DR ROSS: But it is over-the-counter. Supplements are something that nobody governs, as you know.

PEGGY: Yes.

DR ROSS: And so it costs about the same to take a bad one as a good one.

PEGGY: So take a good one.

DR ROSS: And so take the good one. There are some brands that are more physician friendly, if you will. Orthomolecular's one of them. Thorne is another one that I used that is available on Amazon. You can buy it over the counter.

Thorne brands – these are all companies that have substantiated that what they say is in there, is in there, and that you're going to be able to document you're going to get the results from the supplement.

PEGGY: We're talking about Orthomolecular brand, for which you must go to your physician and say, "I'm interested in this brand."

DR ROSS: Correct.

PEGGY: And Thorne brand. And of these brands, what are the things we're taking? What do we want to take from them?

DR ROSS: So one of the things are the B vitamins, and B vitamins are very important. I like Methyl B vitamins, and so I use Orthomolecular Methyl B-12 that's sublingual. It goes under the tongue.

That way you're taking the G.I. tract out of the picture, because oftentimes people don't absorb things. So just because you can take the pill and you can swallow it, it doesn't mean you're going to benefit from it. So we use sublingual.

PEGGY: And that gets absorbed into the bloodstream so that you're getting the benefit of it. Okay.

DR ROSS: Absolutely. And it bypasses the GI tract – yes. And we use Methyl CPG, a supplement that I use for methylating. It helps people with methylation problems.

PEGGY: Okay.

DR ROSS: And the methylated form is very important, because if you do have the MTHFR gene, you're not able to methylate, so you have to have it methylated for you.

PEGGY: What else might people be able to access that would be helpful?

DR ROSS: I use curcumin.

PEGGY: Curcumin.

DR ROSS: And the curcumin that I use is Enhansa. I honestly believe this is probably one of the best products I've ever used. I've tried other brands, and I have not gotten the same results.

PEGGY: Enhansa curcumin. And what's the dosage that you get – or does that depend upon the exposure that you find?

DR ROSS: It depends on the exposure and the level. But if I feel like I understand where the exposure's come from, I use high doses. So sometimes I will use 3600 mg.

PEGGY: That is a high dose.

DR ROSS: That is.

PEGGY: Curcumin is often recommended as just a good thing to take for your brain. So do you think a lower dose might be appropriate just for people who are interested in their brain health?

DR ROSS: Yes. For people who are just interested in their brain health, the Enhansa comes in 600 mg, and I would recommend 1800.

PEGGY: So taking three pills...

DR ROSS: Correct.

PEGGY: And it's Enhansa.

DR ROSS: Enhansa, yes.

PEGGY: Spell that for us?

DR ROSS: It's E-N-H-A-N-S-A.

PEGGY: We heard about one of your patients who's now driving again, and who's taking care of her family, essentially.

DR ROSS: That's right.

PEGGY: Do you have other stories you can tell us?

DR ROSS: I do, actually. I have my very first patient, who was a nurse practitioner, and her husband's a physician. She is doing so much better that he actually went to see a – I think it was a medical rep that was showing them a new procedure, and she was able to get up and help the rep prepare the procedure and do the whole thing.

PEGGY: And I assume this is something that, no way could she could have done it before.

DR ROSS: No way she could have done it before.

PEGGY: It's an enormous change.

DR ROSS: And she's doing really well. She does what's required – you know, when you're on this protocol, you have to stay on the protocol. That's one thing that Dr. Bredesen has noted – when people deviate or come off of it, their symptoms all come right back.

So this particular patient does really well with IV glutathione, and that's another thing that I really use for these patients where I've seen a big difference.

PEGGY: Okay, that's important. Let's talk about IV glutathione. This is something I think people want to know about.

DR ROSS: Right. I use the glutathione that's made by Wellness Pharmacy, and I think they're the only people that actually have a patent on their glutathione in our country.

I try to use it in all my patients. Sometimes it's hard to set up. My patients come from all over, and the laws vary in different states. But the IV glutathione seems to really help mold patients, because one of the mycotoxins, gliotoxin, actually depletes the glutathione storages.

PEGGY: Okay, just refresh us. What is glutathione doing for you? If it's depleted, what's the problem there?

DR ROSS: Right. Glutathione is our body's strongest antioxidant, and so it's very important for the detox pathways as well. We all need it, and if you have the MTHFR, it's even more important.

What we're finding is a lot of these people have similar genetic problems, such as MTHFR, and such as the HLA susceptibility. So the glutathione is a big part of it.

PEGGY: I'm curious if you've seen any evidence of a kind of before-and-after nature in brain images, like for instance, with this woman you're telling me about.

DR ROSS: Absolutely. She's actually scheduled to have her imaging redone, and I think that it will probably be astounding. I have a feeling.

PEGGY: What was she like before?

DR ROSS: She was in the 1% for hippocampal volume. And we also do a MoCA study on these patients, which is the Montreal Cognitive Assessment. Initially she was a 10, and now she's up to 22.

PEGGY: Wow.

DR ROSS: It goes up to 30, so she's doing very well.

PEGGY: 1% of hippocampal, so that's... hippocampal volume refers to the section of the brain that's the hippocampus, where your short-term memory is.

DR ROSS: That's right.

PEGGY: And it's where Alzheimer's initially strikes. So 1% means that of the population, she had a

1% volume, meaning it had shrunk, that she had such a shrunken section of the brain. And this had been activated by the mold.

DR ROSS: I believe that that was a big part of it. I think there are probably numerous factors, but...

PEGGY: Well, you mentioned a time of life when your hormones are changing.

DR ROSS: Right. I think it makes us more vulnerable. She also was using a nasal spray called VIP, which is compounded. The studies have shown that VIP spray will increase the hippocampal volume. It's something that we use in patients. We use it very carefully. We're cautious, because the FDA is looking at it at this point in time to determine its safety, and I think there have been a few issues.

However, having said that, when you have a very low hippocampal volume, VIP spray is something that has proven to increase the hippocampal volume. It's something that we do use.

PEGGY: And how do we get this? Do we just go to our local chain store pharmacy?

DR ROSS: No, no, this is compounded, and there's a handful of pharmacies that actually are more biotoxin-type pharmacies. I get this from Hopkinton in Hopkinton, Massachusetts.

PEGGY: Hopkinton?

DR ROSS: Hopkinton Pharmacy.

PEGGY: And that's something we could do online? We could go there and call them?

DR ROSS: A physician would have to order it.

PEGGY: Okay, compounding means that it's specially made.

DR ROSS: It's specially made, correct.

PEGGY: And the physician orders it. But now you know to ask your physician for this.

DR ROSS: That's right.

PEGGY: Okay. What else can we do for people who are not detoxing well, and that's helping to bring on this horrible brain response? How can we help them detox?

DR ROSS: In my practice we use infrared sauna, because you have to think about all the different ways that our body detoxes, and sweating is very important. I find oftentimes that people who are very toxic are poor sweaters. They don't sweat.

PEGGY: What's an infrared sauna?

DR ROSS: An infrared sauna uses infrared wavelength that actually increases heat in your body, and it helps you to detox. It's kind of a dry sauna. They're very, very comfortable. People get in and they relax. They love it.

PEGGY: Are they expensive to buy?

DR ROSS: There are varying degrees, or different types. You can actually get a portable one that you can take with you.

PEGGY: Wow.

DR ROSS: And I think it's probably about $1200, and you can get a larger one. We have an infrared sauna that seats three people. Now, we never put three people in there, but it gives you a little bit of room. It actually has Bluetooth. You can listen to music, and you can relax. People love it. They feel like they really can get in there and relax, and a lot of my patients will buy these as well.

PEGGY: So these are ways that you can help your body detox if you've been exposed to mold, but we want to go back to the first principle, which is, you do have to get yourself out of the mold environment.

DR ROSS: That's probably one of the most difficult parts, because if you think about it, we all have a house, and when your house has mold, it's a very difficult thing to come to grips with. You have to end up leaving, and oftentimes leave everything that you own in it, or when you take it with you, you will cross-contaminate the place you move to.

PEGGY: So – everything you own. That means your furniture, your clothes, your books, your papers, your...

DR ROSS: That's right.

PEGGY: The different types of Alzheimer's that Dr. Bredesen has identified... maybe take us through those. Which are the most common? Is this really very common as a cause of Alzheimer's?

DR ROSS: That's an interesting question, because when Dr. Bredesen first started doing his studying, he felt that this would probably be about 15% of the population.

PEGGY: One-five.

DR ROSS: And now we are realizing it's about 70%, and it may even be more. That's part of the study that we're looking at. Because we're realizing that these markers, these inflammatory markers that we look at, which he thought would be in a very small group of people, are in a great many, and at this point we think it's about 70%.

PEGGY: Just to clarify, when we say 70%, it's not 70% of the population, but 70% of the population presenting with Alzheimer's.

DR ROSS: Yes, that's correct.

PEGGY: So this may be the most significant factor.

DR ROSS: It may be a very large factor. There also was a recent study done that revealed that they believe that it also stems from pollution, environmental pollution. If you think about it, that, too, may evoke the same response in the body. So we're looking at this very closely right now.

PEGGY: Well, that would fit in with inhalational, right? You're breathing in air that might have toxins. Are there other biotoxins, other than mold, that are common that we should know about?

DR ROSS: Absolutely. Lyme disease is a biotoxin. The spirochete Borrelia burgdorferi, which causes Lyme, is a biotoxin. Dinoflagellates in the ocean are biotoxins. It's like a living toxin.

PEGGY: In the ocean – so if you swim, you might get exposure to this? Is that right?

DR ROSS: If you are someone who works on the water, you could be exposed in that fashion. I suppose swimming as well. Certainly, when you hear of towns or the ocean having a red tide, and towns that are on the water right there, there have been episodes where people develop fibromyalgia and chronic fatigue. It's sort of a mysterious illness in the town, and it would be related to the red tide.

PEGGY: Okay, so if it's from water, obviously, it's not inhalational.

DR ROSS: Well actually, we don't know. We think the toxins may be airborne.

PEGGY: Oh, the toxins in the water...

DR ROSS: ...from the red tide...

PEGGY: ...that release spores, or something like that?

DR ROSS: That's right.

PEGGY: Oh, it's so creepy. It's just very, very creepy.

DR ROSS: That's right.

PEGGY: Okay. Probably Lyme is so common. People may have both. They may have multiple factors, including Lyme.

DR ROSS: That's correct. Well, there's a multi-susceptible gene that actually occurs in one percent of the population, and oftentimes we'll find that they have both.

PEGGY: They have both, okay. What's a timeline? If you do everything right... if, let's say, you tell the patient, "Oh-oh, you've got mold," the next day they leave their home. I mean, under ideal circumstances here that you can just figure out the logistics. How soon are you going to get better? What are you seeing?

DR ROSS: We're seeing that anything you see with an Alzheimer's patient that appears to be positive is a great sign of things to come in the future. Probably six months to a year is really a good rule of thumb to look for.

PEGGY: So it's not something, unfortunately, that just turns around. You take the curcumin, and you take the Brain Octane, and you know...

DR ROSS: Well, I think you start to see changes in about a month.

PEGGY: Okay.

DR ROSS: It's very subtle, very small, but I think it takes a good six months to really see things turning around, and that's using the whole protocol. That's doing your brain exercises.

PEGGY: Okay, brain exercises. What does that mean? What are brain exercises?

DR ROSS: It's an app that you can get on your phone, and they're little brain exercises that you can work on, and they will develop your memory and help with the cognitive function. We encourage our patients to do this daily, and oftentimes in the beginning they don't enjoy it, and I always have to remind them that we're trying, you know, we're really accentuating your weakness here, and nobody wants to feel...

PEGGY: Right.

DR ROSS: But that's how you're going to get stronger, and that helps tremendously.

We also work on exercising the body. We want them to do more cardiovascular work, and sometimes recommend doing little sprints here and there. I actually have a patient who gets up in the morning, does 1500 jumping jacks, and if she doesn't do that, she jumps rope. But she feels like it clears her brain.

PEGGY: 1500 jumping jacks.

DR ROSS: She can tell a difference.

PEGGY: Wow.

DR ROSS: So that's increasing the BDNF in her brain, which is the hormone.

PEGGY: And just tell us what that is.

DR ROSS: That's basically your brain's hormone. It helps with your cognitive function.

We also use a high-fat diet. The diet that I've been using is the Mito Diet through the Institute for Functional Medicine, and that feeds your mitochondria, which are your cells' little powerhouses. That's where we get our energy. And our brain is a very rich mitochondrial environment.

PEGGY: I haven't heard the term "Mito Diet" before.

DR ROSS: So the Mito Diet – it's IFM's way of packaging a high-fat diet, and it is designed for people with Alzheimer's disease, also people with Parkinson's disease.

PEGGY: Important to know. How can we find this? Can we go online?

DR ROSS: You can absolutely go online, and Google it, and you should be able to find it.

PEGGY: M-I-T-O?

DR ROSS: M-I-T-O, Mito Diet, from IFM.

PEGGY: Okay, from the Institute for Functional Medicine.

DR ROSS: That's correct.

PEGGY: So you want the Mito Diet that's going to be high in healthy fats, and it's going to stimulate the mitochondria in your cells to produce more cellular energy going in your brain.

DR ROSS: Absolutely.

PEGGY: Okay, that sounds good. So okay, now we've got people. They're doing 1500 jumping jacks.

They're doing their other things – how are they going to have time for anything else? They're doing that. They're on their phone app, doing the brain exercise...

DR ROSS: That's right. The brain exercises. And they're eating. They're eating properly.

PEGGY: And they're eating. You're cooking your healthy food. I think this does raise the issue that if you're going to get better, it's a commitment .

DR ROSS: It's a commitment, absolutely, and they need support. Support is very important.

PEGGY: So who does this support come from? Tell me us about support.

DR ROSS: We have a lot of amazing husbands. Because really and truly, I see more women than I do men.

PEGGY: Why is that? Is that because of menopause, as you were saying, that they're more vulnerable?

DR ROSS: I'm wondering. I don't really understand it, but I do see more...

PEGGY: Are the women more in the home environment, where they're more exposed?

DR ROSS: That's a very good question. A lot of them, though, had careers. It does concern me. When they become ill, they spend more time at home, and I think that then things deteriorate quickly.

PEGGY: Oh, I see, because they're locked into that mold environment.

DR ROSS: That's right.

PEGGY: Okay, so what are the husbands doing to help them?

DR ROSS: These husbands will get up in the morning before they go to work, and they will set up the whole protocol, which entails putting out the supplements. Oftentimes people will be on many different pills. They will have their cholestyramine, and then they'll encourage their spouse to get up and exercise before they leave. They will oftentimes do brain games with them as well, to work on the brain HQ.

And then the other thing that is a part of this protocol is mindfulness training. It requires them to meditate and work on stress reduction, and sometimes that's a really difficult thing.

Some people are better at it than others, and so we find that the spouses do all of this with their wives, or also their wives do it with their husbands, although as I stated, I have more women than men at this point in time.

The other part of the protocol that's really important is sleep. Sleep is very important. To get eight hours of sleep is a big part. Sometimes that can be challenging.

PEGGY: And how do you help people sleep better?

DR ROSS: We talk about sleep hygiene. It's really important to try and calm yourself down before you get ready to go to bed, kind of tone things down, dim the lights. That can be difficult in a house full of children.

PEGGY: Yes.

DR ROSS: Some of these people have children, and so things take on a different tone, so to speak, than the traditional Alzheimer's patient that is elderly and doesn't have anybody at home.

PEGGY: Yeah, that's, that's really challenging, what you're saying. If you're exposed to toxins, and you have that genetic predisposition, you're developing almost full-blown Alzheimer's at a young age when you want to still be caring for children.

DR ROSS: That's right.

PEGGY: At that level of responsibility, this is a very challenging situation.

DR ROSS: Very challenging.

PEGGY: And then the husband – you're seeing mostly husbands – has to somehow manage everything.

DR ROSS: That's right.

PEGGY: The house, the job, the children...

DR ROSS: And oftentimes their spouse has to leave the house before they can come up with a plan for the house. So they're at home still with the children, trying to determine how do you get the house fixed, and how do you create a safe environment? So it's very challenging.

PEGGY: It's very challenging, but what you're telling us is that there's hope, right?

DR ROSS: Absolutely.

PEGGY: Because I think we should start wrapping things up, let's go back to that score, that MoCA score.

DR ROSS: The MoCA score.

PEGGY: And let's look a little bit at that, and the kind of good results that people can expect if they do what they need to do.

DR ROSS: If they do what they need to do, honestly, we start seeing good things, and so they can develop. Their memory comes back. They're functional, and I think Dr. Bredesen has shown over four years with 100 people that they've all been reversed, for the most part. I think 90% have been reversed, and some have gone back to work. Some people don't want their names given because...

PEGGY: They're at work.

DR ROSS: Yeah, they're at work and they don't want their employers to know, I think. But it's very empowering to know you can do something about this.

PEGGY: Dr. Dale Bredesen, who we've referred to a lot, and who I have interviewed, is actually reversing this in nine out of 10 patients, and training physicians like you. So more and more physicians are going to have this knowledge, and hopefully be dispersed throughout the country, so that people can access a doctor who's going to help them with this. That's what's coming.

In the meantime, if somebody's watching this, and they think that this kind of approach would be helpful, how do they search for a doctor?

DR ROSS: I would encourage them to go online to DrBredesen.com, and they will be able to get a list of physicians in their area who have been trained in this protocol.

PEGGY: And that's very important to know. There is help. And would it be a good idea to go to the Functional Medicine website? Is that also a good plan?

DR ROSS: I don't know that IFM at this point differentiates physicians that have trained through the Bredesen protocol.

PEGGY: Okay.

DR ROSS: They are doing the training. They have taken that over, but I don't know that that information is available on their website.

PEGGY: Okay, so we're going to go to Dr. Bredesen's website, and if we do this... if we find a doctor, and if we commit to this program... just help us understand that there's a realistic cause for optimism, because these families are dealing with a whole lot of problems here. Let's give them some optimism.

DR ROSS: I definitely think there's hope, and I think that they can definitely see things change for the good. In my own patient I've seen changes, for example, changes that I can follow, and measurable changes on the MoCA test.

PEGGY: The MoCA, the cognitive...

DR ROSS: The Montreal Cognitive Assessment. I can see changes in my patient. So she's gone from a 10 to a 22, and that's huge. And that means that she's now functioning. I'm not sure that you would realize she has Alzheimer's if she were in the room with us.

PEGGY: So it really, essentially, boils down to that: Do you function or not? Can you live your life or not? Is your family totally wrapped up in caring for you, or is everybody free to go about their business, because you're self-sufficient?

DR ROSS: That's right. That's right.

PEGGY: This is big stuff.

DR ROSS: Oh, it's huge. It's absolutely huge.

PEGGY: Okay. Well, thank you so much, Dr. Ross, for sharing this absolutely life-saving information with us, information we're really not going to find many other places.

And thank you for watching, and I hope that you've gained some insight in the show about the possibility that symptoms that may seem mysterious and that may be powerfully affecting cognition, may, in fact, originate from mold and from other toxins, and that there are things you can do about it. You can be tested for it. You can treat it, and you can, in fact, get better. So thank you very much.

Interview with Pamela Wartian Smith, M.D., M.P.H.

PEGGY SARLIN: Hello, I'm Peggy Sarlin, and today I'm in Grosse Pointe, Michigan, where I have the pleasure of speaking with Dr. Pamela Wartian Smith, who is going to tell you exactly how you can figure out what is causing your memory problem.

Dr. Smith is the author of an excellent book. I have it here. It's called *What You Must Know About Memory Loss and How You Can Stop It*, and she is a diplomate of the American Academy of Anti-Aging Physicians.

She's the owner and the Director of the Center for Personalized Medicine, and she is a well-known authority on wellness and anti-aging. So welcome, Dr. Smith.

DR PAMELA WARTIAN SMITH: Thank you very much.

PEGGY: So Dr. Smith, let's begin by talking about what your goal is if a patient comes to you with any kind of a memory issue. What's your ultimate goal when you treat them?

DR SMITH: Our goal is to look at the cause of the problem, and not just treat symptoms, and to develop a very customized and personalized approach for every single patient.

PEGGY: Well, that's why you do personalized medicine. Now I get the title.

So the fact that you want to get to the root cause is a little bit different, because many times we see doctors treating symptoms, and not going deeper into finding out what's causing these symptoms.

DR SMITH: That's really the good news in medicine in 2016 and beyond. We really can look at the cause of many disease processes, including cognitive decline.

PEGGY: Okay, so how are we going to do that? Somebody comes in either for themselves, or maybe they bring their spouse, or they bring a parent. And something is going wrong with this person, maybe even seriously wrong. What's your checklist for figuring out the source of the problem?

DR SMITH: Most kinds of memory loss are inflammatory in nature. Inflammation's good if there's a small amount, because it helps you heal. But too much will cause a problem in any place in the body, including the brain.

So we do look at causes of inflammation. They can be hormonal, as in hormonal imbalance. They can be related to heavy metals. There are many different avenues.

Memory loss really is a multi-factorial problem, and so we just go down the road of looking at each of these in a very customized approach.

PEGGY: It's interesting that you say it's multi-factored, and that means that the answer might involve many different factors, rather than looking for the single magic pill that's going to do everything for you. You're going to come at it from several angles.

DR SMITH: We are. For example, if we're looking at women or men, we do know that hormonal function has a lot to do with memory. For example, for men, testosterone literally equals memory. So if testosterone has started to decline, we want to measure it and replace it appropriately.

The same thing for women. Estrogen equals memory, so we measure and replace appropriately with the right kinds of estrogens. There's even a hormone of memory, and it's called pregnenolone. Have you ever heard of that hormone?

PEGGY: Well, I have. I read a lot about memory and the brain, but most people haven't. I think most people know estrogen and testosterone, but they don't know... okay. You pronounce it for me.

DR SMITH: It's so funny to me that the hormone of memory would be hard to say – pregnenolone –

PEGGY: Pregnenolone.

DR SMITH: And hard to spell. It's – to me, it's –

PEGGY: Hard to remember.

DR SMITH: It is hard to remember.

PEGGY: It's hard to remember. But what does it do for us?

DR SMITH: It's the mother hormone. It actually makes estrogen, progesterone, testosterone, DHEA and cortisol, our hormone of stress. And stress plays a very large role when it comes to memory. Whether you had stress as a child... stress when you're 30... stress when you're 60 – that all plays a role.

We can measure your stress hormone, cortisol. It is a salivary test, and if cortisol is not normal, the good news is we can normalize it and balance it in every single person.

PEGGY: That's tremendous news you're bringing us. Just to review for a minute, let's go back to cortisol. Cortisol is the stress hormone, and you can measure it. It's a saliva test – that's not too scary. You spit into a cup or something like that. And you can solve the problem of too much cortisol. So how do you do that? How do you balance it?

DR SMITH: When you're first stressed, cortisol elevates. When you stay stressed for a long time, it becomes too low. You have to have cortisol to live. If you don't have cortisol you die in seven days.

PEGGY: Seven days.

DR SMITH: In seven days.

PEGGY: Oh.

DR SMITH: So it's a must for living. The body will make cortisol above all those other hormones.

For example, you could be 37. Your pregnenolone level, the hormone of memory, could be five, which is very low, due to stress. And if stress is the cause of the problem, we want to deal with that hormone.

When cortisol's not normal, cholesterol can go up, blood pressure can go up, blood sugar can go up, the immune system becomes compromised. Thyroid hormones, the hormones that regulate everything in the entire body, may dysfunction. People put on weight... and stress – I mean, who isn't stressed in today's society?

So we measure cortisol in everyone. It's a great place to begin for any disease process, but particularly for memory.

PEGGY: Very, very interesting to know. So somebody comes in, let's say, and they're experiencing memory problems. You measure their cortisol, and what do you – let's say something's wrong. From what you were saying, it sounded like either it might be too high, or too low. You might see either one.

DR SMITH: Correct.

PEGGY: Now what are you going to do?

DR SMITH: Well, first of all, we put people on a multivitamin, a good pharmaceutical grade one if they're not on a pharmaceutical grade vitamin, because the adrenal glands – the glands that sit above your kidneys that make cortisol – need basic nutrients that are in a multivitamin.

Of course, we want people to eat well. But as we age, the body makes less of some nutrients, so we begin with a multivitamin.

PEGGY: Could I just stop you there? You said "pharmaceutical grade." Does that mean prescription? Is that what it means?

DR SMITH: It doesn't. But what it means is two things: pharmaceutical grade is when the nutrient is guaranteed to be 100% pure, as proven with outside verification, and it's also what we call "bioavailable," meaning that it gets into your body, and it does what it is supposed to do.

PEGGY: Right. Do you recommend specific brands? Is that something you could feel comfortable doing, or do people choose their own source?

DR SMITH: We do recommend great brands. The brands we recommend have clinically-controlled trials that actually show us that the nutrients get into the body and do what they're supposed to do.

Three main nutrients decline with age, starting at about the age of 50: Coenzyme Q10, alpha lipoic acid, and L-carnitine. All of those nutrients are fueling sources for the body, including the brain.

They're all very important for cognition. We can go back and measure them, but they need basic nutrients to make them.

Also when it comes to stress, we give adaptogenic herbs – herbs that help the body deal with life. Ashwagandha, ginseng, rhodiola are some great adaptogenic herbs, which means they work if cortisol's too high or too low.

PEGGY: This is an important point, I think, for people to understand. It's adaptogenic because it's going to help your body adapt, whether too high, too low... It's a tonic.

DR SMITH: It is a tonic. And it's so important that people also understand that cortisol takes a long time to balance.

PEGGY: Ah!

DR SMITH: When it comes to pregnenolone, within 90 days we can usually balance that. But if people are really stressed it takes one to two years to normalize cortisol.

PEGGY: Oh, whoa! That's a lot of time.

DR SMITH: It is. But stress reduction techniques are also important – prayer, meditation, Tai Chi, yoga, Qigong, exercise, massage, breathing techniques. Even if a busy person says they have no time to do stress reduction techniques, they can sit at their desk and take deep breaths and let them out. That's a great stress reducer for today's world.

PEGGY: And if you reduce your stress, this is going to help bring back your mother hormone that you mentioned, the – see, I can't remember the name of what it is!

DR SMITH: It really is funny, that name, pregnenolone, isn't it?

PEGGY: Yes, it is, pregnenolone. You'll see results sooner in terms of that hormone than the cortisol. The cortisol's going to take a longer time to find the proper balance.

DR SMITH: It does, but we can help balance it.

The other thing about cortisol that's really important is that it affects blood sugar and the hormone insulin. And the research worldwide now, when we look at memory loss, is focusing on the hormone insulin. There are insulin receptors in your brain, and as a result, if you have too much insulin or too little, it can negatively impact your memory.

PEGGY: Well, this brings up the topic, usually, of what to eat. When you're talking about insulin, you're often talking about food and healthy diet. Is there a recommendation you make to your patients? Is there an across-the-board recommendation, or do you tailor it to individual people?

DR SMITH: Really, both. If we're going to make an across-the-board recommendation, then we usually recommend the Mediterranean diet, because it's anti-inflammatory, and it works well for most people.

But the science is now here to do genetic testing, where we can literally measure your genomes and see what's on them, and tailor-make an eating program for you.

PEGGY: Wow.

DR SMITH: And exercise, because exercise maintains memory. We can do genome testing. When I did my own, it was really very fascinating.

I do not have what's called the "sprinter gene." If you have the sprinter gene, exercising will help you maintain your weight. I don't have that gene, so I can exercise every single day and it will not affect my weight. But what I exercise for is to maintain memory.

I was really lucky. I got to meet Jack LaLanne before he passed away. So I said, "Hey, Jack, how do I learn to like exercise?" Because I truly do not like it. I do not get the high that some people get from it.

He told me the most amazing thing: "I don't like exercise either, but I love the results."

PEGGY: He didn't – Jack LaLanne did not like exercise?

DR SMITH: He did not like exercise.

PEGGY: Well, there's certainly a man who compensated. Okay.

DR SMITH: He did, but it maintains memory, and it doesn't have to be pumping iron to maintain memory. Studies have shown that things like ballroom dancing are great exercise and help maintain cognition.

PEGGY: I'm going back to what you said about the gene analysis. You're saying now – this is totally new to me – you can get genetic testing that says, "Oh, this is the right exercise program for you."

DR SMITH: Yes. And the same thing for how you eat. It's actually on a gene, and sometimes people have something called a "SNIP," a single nucleotide polymorphism. You can just call it SNIP.

PEGGY: That's easier, okay.

DR SMITH: It is much easier, and it determines our taste, whether we can taste bitter or sweet. It determines our cravings. For example, some people have sugar cravings they have a hard time turning off. It determines a whole battery of things, whether we get inflammation from the foods we eat – all of that can be tested now with genomic testing.

PEGGY: How new is this? I mean, this is really new, isn't it?

DR SMITH: It's very new, and in our personal practice we've been doing it for four years now.

PEGGY: I see. The idea that you can figure out from your exact genetic testing, "This is the right diet for my body. This is the right exercise program for my body" – it's just extremely exciting!

DR SMITH: It is, because when it comes to memory, there are really five things that are important.

PEGGY: Okay.

DR SMITH: One, how you eat, and nobody eats perfect.

PEGGY: But you have to eat right most of the time.

DR SMITH: Correct.

PEGGY: Not all of the time.

DR SMITH: It's that 80/20 rule, or 90/10 rule. I happen to have a sweet tooth, personally, so every Sunday afternoon I have something sweet. But I don't eat sweets every day. This last week, my Sunday treat was a hot fudge sundae.

PEGGY: But it was on Sunday, and that was it for the week.

DR SMITH: That's all I ate for the week.

PEGGY: Right.

DR SMITH: Now, the week before that I cheated slightly, because it was my birthday.

PEGGY: Oh.

DR SMITH: So I had two things.

PEGGY: Okay, Happy Birthday!

DR SMITH: Thank you. But eating right is really important. Exercise is important to maintain memory.

PEGGY: Let's talk about exercise, because this is a new idea, that our bodies are genetically programmed to respond in different ways... what works for somebody else may not work for you.

You hear a lot of different advice about types of exercise – the stretching, the weight bearing, the cardiovascular, aerobic – whatever. What's the minimum for people who want to maintain their memory and don't like exercise? What's the minimum?

DR SMITH: Well, two studies have been done which are a variety. So again, it's probably personalized. One very recent study showed that if you do advanced cardio – meaning you really do double your pulse for 20 minutes, then once a week is enough.

PEGGY: Oh, once a week. Well, that's good news for people who don't want to exercise much.

DR SMITH: It is. More commonly, the studies have shown three times a week, doubling your pulse for 20 minutes is perfect. Now, it takes a little longer, because you should warm up and cool down, and if people are over the age of 50, we do recommend, before they begin an exercise program, that they see their primary care doctor and have a stress test if they have not been exercising.

PEGGY: And that's because of potential heart issues?

DR SMITH: Absolutely.

PEGGY: If they start suddenly getting on that treadmill and getting into a sweat they could be at risk. All right, you said there were five things about memory, so where are we? We were going to eat right, and we were going to ...?

DR SMITH: Exercise.

PEGGY: We were going to exercise.

DR SMITH: Sleep is key for memory. When you don't have good sleep hygiene, meaning that you don't sleep at least six and a half hours to eight hours a night of good, restorative sleep, it drives up your blood sugar. And it's one of the mechanisms that causes memory loss.

So sleep is important, hormonal balance, and then to be nutritionally sound.

PEGGY: Going back to hormonal balance for a minute, did we completely cover how we were going to bring the cortisol into balance? There were stress reduction techniques. Oh, it was the adaptogenic herbs, things like rhodiola and ashwagandha. Are there tricks there to manage the cortisol problem?

DR SMITH: If people are stressed and wired – because some people are more wired, and we want a nice balance – then we give calming herbs, too, like lemon balm, chamomile. Some people need those, some people do not. It's really all about balance.

PEGGY: I notice when you said you were going to calm people down you were going to give them these natural herbs. You weren't going to give them prescription drugs. You weren't going to give them Xanax, or whatever. Is that correct? Do you even use those drugs in your practice?

DR SMITH: I believe in traditional medicine, so I use almost every single medication that you can imagine and a very personalized approach. But if I can have people eat better, and sleep better, and exercise, and have hormonal balance, and have the right nutrients, many times people don't need medication.

PEGGY: Which is preferable, which is truly preferable. Okay, there were five items. We're eating right. We're exercising. We're balancing our hormones, was that it?

DR SMITH: Mm hm.

PEGGY: Sleep, and stress. Is that all five? Did we cover all five?

DR SMITH: Well, eating right.

PEGGY: Right.

DR SMITH: Okay. Exercise, sleep, hormones, and nutrients.

PEGGY: And nutrients. Now, let's talk about the nutrients. What are the supplements you would recommend? Let's say you're over 50. Are there supplements that you should take on a daily basis, even if you're eating well, just as a neuro-protective thing, just to be good to your brain in the future?

DR SMITH: Well, the perfect answer to that is that we can do a test and measure the level of 37 vitamins in your body. We can measure amino acids, fatty acids, organic acids, which are pathways that help with cognition and the rest of the functions in the body that require nutrients.

But to give you a simpler answer to that, really, everybody should be on a multivitamin.

PEGGY: Okay.

DR SMITH: They should be on a probiotic, good bacteria, for their gut. And they should be on omega-3 fatty acids like fish oil or some other kind of omega-3 fatty acid. That's probably the bare minimum that people should start with.

PEGGY: That's very important to know. That's like basic black in your wardrobe. That's what you need on your kitchen shelf to take every day.

In your book, you have an interesting structure where people can answer questionnaires to try to figure out the source of the problem. You begin with cardiovascular. What are some of the questions you ask people to answer about the cardiovascular system that might affect their memory, so they can start figuring out, "Maybe that's where my problem's coming from"?

DR SMITH: Well, from the viewpoint of heart health or cardiovascular disease, the vessels in your heart are the same kind of vessels that run to your brain. So if you have hardening of the arteries in the heart, you have hardening of the arteries in your brain.

PEGGY: They're connected.

DR SMITH: They are connected. And so heart health equals brain health. Brain health equals heart health. And when we look at cardiovascular issues, particularly for women, sometimes it's a difficult discussion because women usually don't get crushing chest pain – hardly ever – if they have an impending heart attack, or if they have vessels that are clogged.

Women may get nausea. They may get shortness of breath. They may have pain on the right shoulder, and not on the left side of the chest.

So what we try and do is recommend that everybody at 50 have a stress test and an EKG to look at the basics of their heart structure.

Also, when we look at cholesterol, cholesterol is not the only risk factor. One-half of people who have a heart attack have very normal cholesterol, so there are other risk factors to look at.

PEGGY: And what are those?

DR SMITH: One of those is homocysteine. Homocysteine's an amino acid, and if it accumulates in the body, there is an increased risk in heart disease and stroke, depression, breast cancer, prostate cancer, and memory loss.

PEGGY: And what's going to cause those raised levels?

DR SMITH: Some people are born with a gene where they don't break down B vitamins well. B vitamins, particularly B-6, B-12, and folate, lower homocysteine. But people can have that SNIP we were talking about, that single nucleotide polymorphism, where they can take B-6, B-12 and folate, and it does not break down homocysteine.

They will need a more activated form like MTHF, which stands for methylene-tetrahydrofolate, or TMG, which stands for trimethylglycine. That's part of what we call the "methylation pathway." To sum up, it's really important for all of those reasons, including memory, that we normalize homocysteine to between six and eight.

PEGGY: Is this something a regular family doctor would look for? Would they check your levels of homocysteine?

DR SMITH: Probably not at this point. Certainly if you saw a specialist in the field of anti-aging medicine, regenerative functional medicine – any of those – metabolic medicine, then they would look at this. In the future, every doctor will be looking at homocysteine.

PEGGY: But people who are watching this can get into the future now. They know they want to get that test, that that's crucial to understand what your current homocysteine level is, in terms of your cognitive health.

DR SMITH: It's very key. It's a blood study that you can have at any major lab. It is a fasting study, so you fast for eight hours before you go in. But it's readily available, and we can normalize it in everyone.

You also don't want homocysteine to be too low. Too low is not good either. It's all about optimal levels of everything.

PEGGY: Optimal. We're trying to optimize your brain here, and your heart, and your overall wellness. That's the goal.

DR SMITH: C-reactive protein is another marker that we look at for heart health and brain health. It's a marker of inflammation. In fact, many researchers believe that high C-reactive protein is the major risk factor for heart disease.

PEGGY: That is the risk factor. Most people don't even know about it. And if you have a high level of that, chances are the inflammation is in your brain as well, you say.

DR SMITH: It is. And the good news is we can normalize that in everyone.

PEGGY: How do you cool it down? How do you bring down that inflammation of the CRP?

DR SMITH: We want the level to be one or below in the CRP test. If it's slightly high, then we can use anti-inflammatory things like omega-3 fatty acids ...

PEGGY: Okay.

DR SMITH: Or other anti-inflammatories. It's probably how statin drugs work. Statin drugs are also anti-inflammatory. We can use many other things to decrease inflammation, like green tea, three cups of green tea a day would be very helpful. Curcumin, turmeric...there are many anti-inflammatory herbal therapies we can use as well.

PEGGY: So if you take these anti-inflammatory herbs, they're going to cool down CRP, and that's going to show up in your blood test so you'll be able to measure that and see how you're doing, right?

DR SMITH: You can. Let's say your CRP level is three. We'll give you some omega-3 fatty acids in the form of fish oil, probably 3,000 mg would be a great place to start. You can use other omega-3's as well, and that will bring the CRP down to one, usually in about 30 days.

PEGGY: That's good. We like that. That's not like the cortisol, where we're twiddling our thumbs for two years.

DR SMITH: This one's quicker.

PEGGY: Okay.

DR SMITH: Some people have a really high C-reactive protein, so perhaps it might be 28.

PEGGY: Wow! And it's supposed to be one?

DR SMITH: It's supposed to be one.

PEGGY: Yikes. Okay.

DR SMITH: If it's really high, that usually means there is an infection in the blood vessels, so we give a traditional antibiotic to clear up that infection, and then the C-reactive protein goes down.

PEGGY: So when you're looking for cardiovascular problems, these are the tests that you do. You're looking at these biomarkers – the CRP, the homocysteine... What are some other ones?

DR SMITH: We look at fibrinogen, which is a clotting factor. We look at ferritin, which is iron, particularly in men. If iron elevates in men or women, it increases the risk of heart disease, but that issue is more common in men than it is in women.

We can look at other inflammatory markers like TNF alpha, interleukin-6... The good news is they're all blood studies. They're all available at almost every major lab, and we can normalize all of them.

PEGGY: It's very good news, because if, let's say, this is the source of your memory problem, and you take care of it with these not-very-scary-sounding remedies – drinking green tea, taking krill oil, or fish oil, or some of these other things you've mentioned, then we're not only protecting our heart, we're protecting our brain. And we're going to feel better.

DR SMITH: We're going to feel better because, again, it's all about balance.

PEGGY: We're going to feel more in balance. We're physically going to feel more in balance.

DR SMITH: We are.

PEGGY: We're going to have more energy?

DR SMITH: We're going to have more energy. Again, a little bit of inflammation heals. That's why if you fall down and you sprain your ankle, the inflammatory process occurs. The ankle swells. It's part of healing, but you're not supposed to stay inflamed.

PEGGY: Right. Now, another possibility you mentioned in your book for memory problems is that there's been some kind of toxic exposure – heavy metals, or something like that. Can you help us understand how that might manifest, and how you might find that? How you might diagnose it?

DR SMITH: Toxic metals are becoming a more important issue with people worldwide. As to how you diagnose it, it is a urine test, and you take what we call a "provocating agent" beforehand. It's a chelating agent, usually a pill.

You take it about an hour before you do the test, and you collect your urine for 6 to 24 hours. It's very important that you're on a multivitamin for 30 days before you do the test because when you take that chelating agent, it takes the minerals out of your body along with measuring your mercury, and all the other toxins.

PEGGY: Oh, I see. So you're going to be depleted unless you're taking a vitamin.

DR SMITH: Yes. The really new studies are showing that when it comes to diabetes, toxic metals play a major role.

PEGGY: Let's talk about this for a while, because diabetes is such a gigantic issue, and because people who have diabetes are dramatically more at risk of getting Alzheimer's and cognitive problems. This is a whole new way to think about diabetes, I think.

DR SMITH: It is a whole new way. More and more, we measure toxic metals in patients, and we can chelate them out. When we look at chelation, if the toxic metal levels are very high, we do IV. But many people just have a moderate amount, or low, and we can give oral chelation over a number of days to lower the lead, mercury, and other toxic levels like cadmium. They can all negatively impact memory.

But your point is very well taken about diabetes, because sometimes people don't realize there are really three kinds of diabetes. There's Type I, where people don't make insulin at all. There's Type II, which is what 95% of Americans have who have diabetes. In Type II, they make insulin, but it doesn't work effectively in the body.

But now there's Type III diabetes, and that's Alzheimer's disease.

PEGGY: And this is a new way of thinking about Alzheimer's as well.

DR SMITH: It is.

PEGGY: Which is that it's diabetes of the brain.

DR SMITH: It is diabetes of the brain in many ways.

PEGGY: And you're saying that a source of that could be an exposure to metals?

DR SMITH: Yes. A major pilot study was done that actually proved this. So now there's a multi-center trial going on, and the early results of that trial are confirming that, for some people, blood sugar elevation is very much related to toxic metal exposure.

PEGGY: This, I think, is important news, and how can people avoid that exposure? Where are they getting this exposure from?

DR SMITH: It's hard to totally avoid. It may be in their drinking water, so purified water is always the best choice.

PEGGY: Okay.

DR SMITH: They may have toxic metal exposure from their pots and pans. It can come from aluminum cans. I mean, there are many ways people can get toxic, and the body is able to handle some toxins. But the body can become overwhelmed.

We now have the ability to also measure PCBs and dioxins, and look at plastics, meaning phthalates. We can measure all those levels too, now.

PEGGY: And not only measure them, but then you can treat them with chelation? Is that essentially how you'd do that?

DR SMITH: With toxic metals, we use chelation. With PCBs and dioxins, they're doing studies to look at the best ways. Infrared sauna is one of those.

PEGGY: Tell us about infrared sauna.

DR SMITH: Well, infrared sauna is slightly different than what you might think of as a "sauna" in your house. It's a special kind of sauna using infrared rays, and you sit in your sauna either at home, your doctor's office, or a medical spa. Three times a week is a good frequency to have a sauna treatment, but it's done with infrared rays, as opposed to other modalities.

PEGGY: It's not dangerous at all?

DR SMITH: It's not.

PEGGY: It's pretty much risk-free?

DR SMITH: The only time it's not risk free is if you do an infrared sauna and then you jump into cold water.

PEGGY: Oh, okay. So don't do that.

DR SMITH: Don't do that.

PEGGY: Don't do that. These are very new ways of thinking about some extremely common medical issues such as diabetes, you know. To think that it might have come from your aluminum pans, or from your drinking water – from accumulated toxins that have built up over the years. This is new.

DR SMITH: This is new. The studies are brand new, really important, but that doesn't stop the importance of eating a healthy diet, and exercise lowers blood sugar as well. Stress can cause blood sugar to elevate.

Even if you don't have a family history, you can still become insulin resistant or develop diabetes if you put your body in a bad environment.

PEGGY: Let's talk about another subject. You've raised the issue that we're much more sophisticated in looking at our personal genetic structure.

Some people are genetically predisposed to Alzheimer's. It runs in their family, and they have a genetic marker for it. So if they come to you, how do you tell if it really is Alzheimer's?

I have a specific question, which is that it's been an ongoing issue that people have been diagnosed with Alzheimer's, then afterwards, after their death, it's been ascertained they didn't have Alzheimer's at all. So is the imaging better? What's the state today, currently, of figuring out with accuracy if somebody has Alzheimer's?

DR SMITH: It's a diagnosis of exclusion, meaning that we can do a PET scan. We can do a SPECT scan. We can do a functional and traditional MRI that will give us hints. But there's not one particular test that says, "Hi, this is Alzheimer's disease."

PEGGY: I see.

DR SMITH: So it's what we call a "diagnosis of exclusion," where we look at other things that could cause the symptoms the person is having.

PEGGY: Okay, so there still doesn't exist that beautiful, perfect imaging system, or whatever, that's going to tell us, "Yes, in fact, this is Alzheimer's."

DR SMITH: No. On SPECT scan and PET scan you can see changes in the brain that occur with cognitive decline of all varieties, but those same changes can occur due to medications and other things.

PEGGY: Okay, so if somebody comes to you, what is the constellation of symptoms, and biomarkers, etc., that's going to make you say, "Yes, this person, in fact, has Alzheimer's."

DR SMITH: We spend a long time with our patients, and it does take a long time when you're interviewing someone to really see where their memory is. There are traditional tests we can do that are very simple, like, "Here's a drawing. Please reproduce it for me."

PEGGY: Right.

DR SMITH: We can have you count backwards by sevens, starting at 100. Sometimes I just have fun with my patients, and I'll say, "Hey, what's going on in the world of politics today?" Or, "What new thing have you read about recently?"

If they say they never read, then I start worrying, because that's one of the signs of early cognitive decline, when people stop reading because they no longer remember what they just read, and so they just –

PEGGY: Right, so short term memory goes.

DR SMITH: It does.

PEGGY: Just to remember the sentence before is too much.

DR SMITH: It is. So if I say, "Hey, when you were 25, how many books did you read in a year?" And then you say, "Oh, I read ten." And then I'll say, "Well, you're 67. How many books did you read last year?" And you say to me you didn't read many, then I want to look further into what is happening with your memory.

PEGGY: I see. Since there isn't this "magical imagery," you're looking at exclusion. You've ruled out other things, and you're observing them and giving them tests like asking them to count backwards from 100, and different things like this.

Let's say you come to the determination that, yes, this patient has Alzheimer's disease. Let's say, early stage Alzheimer's. How are you going to treat them? How are you going to get them better?

DR SMITH: We want to offer them every modality that's available. So commonly, they are put on a medication to stabilize memory loss. We do measure their hormones, and we optimize them as much as possible.

Studies have shown that testosterone and DHEA and pregnenolone for men, and estrogen, DHEA, and pregnenolone for women can help prevent memory loss, but can also stabilize memory loss. In a couple of studies, they stabilized maybe mild reversal of memory loss, including Alzheimer's disease.

The idea is, how can we stabilize it? Normalizing blood sugar, looking at toxins, are both very important.

There are also infectious causes. You were mentioning earlier that some people were diagnosed, and then they really didn't have Alzheimer's.

PEGGY: Right.

DR SMITH: A big one now is Lyme disease.

PEGGY: Lyme disease, yes.

DR SMITH: Lyme disease is huge. It can affect the brain and cognition. If we go back and treat that, then we may be able to retrieve some of the memory. Parasitic infections are a factor. It is globalization of the world. People travel everywhere.

PEGGY: And they come back with parasites.

DR SMITH: They do. And then the parasites can invade the brain as well. We give them an anti-parasitic agent, good bacteria... Those kind of things are reversible causes of cognitive decline, commonly.

PEGGY: And I think it's fair to say that people can have more than one thing wrong with them at the same time.

Again, the approach of coming at it from multiple angles. There's so much to think about here. We've learned so much from you. Does anybody spring to mind, a story of somebody that you've helped, a case where you've seen their memory come back, and their cognitive function – someone who made a really good recovery?

DR SMITH: Yes. One of them is my patient Sally, and she allows me to tell the story because she's so thrilled about it.

When Sally came in to see me, she had an 8 am appointment, and she showed up at 12:00 noon.

EGGY: Oops!

DR SMITH: She lived four blocks from this office – four blocks, and she couldn't find her way here.

PEGGY: Oh, she couldn't find –

DR SMITH: For four hours.

PEGGY: That sounds like Alzheimer's. I mean, one of the first things you lose is your sense of spatial orientation.

DR SMITH: It does. It sounds just like Alzheimer's disease, and the reason she was coming to our practice is that her doctor noticed she had some memory loss.

And so she came in to see us, and we ended up decreasing inflammation. We normalized her blood sugar. We optimized function of her thyroid, which regulates all the hormones in the body, and everything else.

She ended up being low in estrogen, progesterone, testosterone, DHEA, and pregnenolone. We optimized all of those, and within about an eight-month period of time, not only could she find her way to the office, but she ended up opening a restaurant with her son who was a world-class chef, which is a five-star restaurant.

PEGGY: Whoa!

DR SMITH: Yes!

PEGGY: I like that punch line! How old was Sally?

DR SMITH: Sally was 67 when she came to see us.

PEGGY: And how old is she now?

DR SMITH: Sally is now, oh gosh, she's almost 80, just shy of 80.

PEGGY: I need a moment to process. When she was 67, she couldn't find her way four blocks here. She's now 80, and opening up five-star restaurants.

DR SMITH: And her husband died many years ago. She has a gentleman friend she travels around the world with.

PEGGY: We should all live as well as Sally! Sounds good.

Well, I want to thank you so much, Dr. Smith, for sharing this really remarkable information. There are so many nuggets here, and there's so much news. There's a lot to think over.

And thank you for watching, and I hope you learned from Dr. Smith. I hope you read her excellent book, which, again, is called *What You Must Know About Memory Loss, and How You Can Stop It*. And I hope you found new avenues to explore how to protect your brain and how to regain memory that you may have lost. So thank you.

Interview with Mary Newport, M.D.

PEGGY SARLIN: Hello, I'm Peggy Sarlin, and today I'm speaking with Dr. Mary Newport in Spring Hill, FL, about how coconut oil can super-fuel your brain. Dr. Newport is a pediatrician and neonatologist who discovered that coconut oil dramatically improved her husband's Alzheimer's, and she has become a determined public advocate of coconut oil as a super fuel for the brain.

She's written two books on the subject, and is really an expert on the practical use of coconut oil in your daily diet. So welcome, Dr. Newport.

DR NEWPORT: Thank you so much, Peggy, for helping me to spread the message.

PEGGY: Now, why coconut oil? For people who, let's say, may be experiencing senior moments, not as sharp as they used to be, feeling forgetfulness, memory loss, confusion... why coconut oil?

DR NEWPORT: Well, coconut oil contains medium chain fatty acids. About 60% of the fats are medium chains, and medium chains when they're consumed are converted partly to ketones, which serve as an alternative fuel for the brain.

And that is important in Alzheimer's disease because it is a type of diabetes of the brain. This may not be widely known. People know about plaques and amyls in the brain, but another very important aspect is that there's a problem with insulin resistance and insulin deficiency in the brain, very much like Type II diabetes, where there is a problem of getting glucose into brain cells in the areas that are affected by Alzheimer's.

PEGGY: So for a person who doesn't have Alzheimer's, a person who is just maybe getting a little bit older, getting a little bit forgetful... might they be in a pre-Alzheimer's state? Might coconut oil in some way prevent the Alzheimer's from ever developing? Or, what is the impact for people, let's say, in their 50's, and 60's, and...?

DR NEWPORT: Yeah, that is the hope. The process of developing insulin resistance and insulin deficiency happens as early as 10 or 20 years before the onset of Alzheimer's – maybe even sooner. It begins happening before a person begins to have symptoms.

There have been studies of young adults in their 20's who are at risk for Alzheimer's by virtue of their family history in which the studies show they already have decreased glucose uptake in those areas of the brain.

So potentially, you would want to prevent the disease, and if you can provide an alternative fuel to the brain to glucose to make up some of that deficit of energy in the brain that you have when you're at risk, you could potentially prevent Alzheimer's disease.

PEGGY: So one aspect of taking coconut oil for your brain is potentially prevention – that you're providing fuel to your brain, and keeping the brain cells well-nourished so they're not going to die off, and you're not going to develop Alzheimer's. That's a long-term goal, which is fabulous.

What about short term? If today I can't remember where I left my glasses, or I can't remember, "What the heck is his name?" – is coconut oil going to help me on a more short-term basis?

DR NEWPORT: I've heard from many people that say yes, that that is the case, that they feel sharper when they take it. People who consider themselves having "brain fog," as they call it.

PEGGY: Brain fog, right. Common complaint.

DR NEWPORT: Yeah. There is a little bit of memory problem, trouble retaining information, reading comprehension and those kinds of things sometimes seem to get –

PEGGY: The focus...

DR NEWPORT: As you age, there's something called "age-related memory impairment" that's not Alzheimer's disease, but it's still the case that your brain isn't using glucose as effectively as it did when you were a young adult.

The people who developed the medical food Axona, which is MCT (medium chain triglycerides) oil, did studies with age-related memory impairment, and they found that just as with Alzheimer's there was improvement in almost half the people that took MCT oil.

And as you and I know, MCT oil is extracted from coconut oil. It's about 60% coconut oil, so potentially, by incorporating coconut oil into your everyday diet and/or using MCT oil in your diet you could bring about some improvement in your memory, and those senior moments or brain fog may improve.

PEGGY: So if you're having brain fog, senior moments, whatever, it potentially means you're moving towards Alzheimer's. That is a real possibility.

DR NEWPORT: It's a possibility.

PEGGY: And one factor could be that your brain is not processing glucose.

DR NEWPORT: Right.

PEGGY: And so by incorporating coconut oil into your diet, you're going to... Okay, explain to us, what does that do for us in terms of fueling the brain?

DR NEWPORT: When you ingest coconut oil, 60% of that is medium chain triglycerides. Your liver converts part of the medium chain triglycerides, or MCT's, to ketone bodies. And ketones easily cross the blood-brain barrier, and they supply an alternative fuel to the brain.

An example of another time that this happens is during starvation or fasting. Usually within 36 or 48 hours, you use up the glucose that's stored in your body, and you can tap into your fat. And when fat is broken down, fatty acids nourish the rest of the body besides the brain, but don't cross into the brain.

But the liver converts some fatty acids to ketones, and the ketones are taken up by the brain. The brain can very easily switch over from using glucose to ketone bodies as an alternative fuel. So that's really how coconut oil works as an alternative fuel to the brain.

PEGGY: It's an alternative fuel to the brain. So we can understand that if our brain is not working as efficiently at using glucose as fuel, we can fuel it up in this other way that can, in fact, taste delicious, too.

DR NEWPORT: Right.

PEGGY: So we'll get into that, because there are many ways that are delicious to keep our brain going, and to prevent future damage. Now, your husband Steve responded very dramatically to coconut oil – within a few hours.

DR NEWPORT: Right.

PEGGY: His brain responded to coconut oil.

DR NEWPORT: Right.

PEGGY: He had Alzheimer's?

DR NEWPORT: He had Alzheimer's. He was 51 – early onset Alzheimer's. He was only 51 years old when he began having problems. He was an accountant. He worked at home for my practice, and began having trouble remembering if he'd been to the bank and the post office, made payroll mistakes, started procrastinating on tax returns...

That's how we discovered he had a problem. But it became progressively worse to the point where, by 2008, when we started using coconut oil, he could no longer even turn on a computer, much less use a calculator or do simple math.

So by 2008 Steve was really on a downward spiral, and we were looking for clinical trials. And I came upon a press release for a medical food. It turned out to be MCT oil, which was converted to ketones. And Steve responded very dramatically the very first time we gave him coconut oil. He had a marked improvement in a Mini Mental Status Exam, a four point improvement from the day before, and thanks to that he actually qualified to participate in a clinical trial.

And then we saw ongoing improvements. His personality returned, his sense of humor. Tremors in his jaw and in his hand subsided. His gait improved. He had a visual disturbance that improved over several months. It was an ongoing response. It was immediate, but then the improvements continued over a period of nearly a year. It was a very dramatic thing for us. So I started getting the message out, and then it evolved into what we're going to talk about.

PEGGY: Well, I understand that we can even see visual evidence of that, because a standard test for Alzheimer's is drawing a clock. And you have drawings of his showing his improvement over a short period of time.

DR NEWPORT: Yeah, it was very fortunate that he just happened to be trying for clinical trials. I wouldn't know about it to start with. I was researching the two drugs that were being tested in the trials when I came upon the medical food that was going to be available a year later.

But he drew a clock face the day before he started coconut oil, and it had just a few little circles, and a few numbers. It was not organized. It was such that the doctor said he was on the verge of severe Alzheimer's.

Two weeks later, after starting coconut oil, he was able to draw a full circle. It had all the numbers in the correct order, and he had a lot of spokes in the clock. I think they were the hands of the clock, but considerable improvement. And then subsequently, he drew even better and better clocks. So that was just a little bit of objective evidence.

PEGGY: Yes, visual evidence that...

DR NEWPORT: Visual evidence that he had improved, but among many other improvements that we were seeing. Steve responded to it very dramatically. Not everybody does quite that dramatically. In some people, the improvements are more obvious after a month or two, or three.

PEGGY: Right. Everybody –

DR NEWPORT: Everybody's different.

PEGGY: Everybody responds according to their unique body.

DR NEWPORT: Right.

PEGGY: So you became very interested and a passionate advocate on behalf of coconut oil with the idea of helping people incorporate coconut oil into their diet on a daily basis. And the idea is that this should be consumed steadily throughout the day? Can you help us understand, what's our objective here? What are we aiming for?

DR NEWPORT: Yes. The objective is to provide ketones as an alternative fuel to the brain, 24/7 if at all possible. In the very beginning I was giving Steve, for breakfast, a measured dose of coconut oil, and then eventually added measured doses at dinner, and at lunch, and then before bedtime, really, with the idea of trying to sustain the ketone levels.

And this was based on actual blood levels being measured – you know, where we could see his level of ketones would peak at about three hours, and then subside over another six or seven hours with coconut oil.

With MCT oil, his level peaked at 90 minutes, and the ketones were gone by three hours. So I actually started mixing the two. I still cook with basic, straight coconut oil, but for other foods, like putting it in salads or in smoothies and that kind of thing, I started mixing MCT and coconut oil together to try to get the best properties of both, so we could get higher levels of ketones and more sustained levels from coconut oil.

If you give it several times a day, you could potentially keep the ketones elevated over a 24-hour period.

PEGGY: So if somebody's starting to get, as we said, senior moments, and brain fog, and all these things... If they eat in a way that's going to keep up their ketone levels and keep their brain nice and nourished with fabulous ketones as an alternative fuel to glucose throughout the day, they can start feeling cognitively sharper.

DR NEWPORT: Right.

PEGGY: So, you have a beautiful show-and-tell here of different products. How are we going to...? Let's begin with coconut oil.

DR NEWPORT: Okay. This is your basic, organic coconut oil, and any coconut oil can be used – it doesn't have to be organic. It can be refined, non-organic coconut oil. It will produce the same effect of raising ketones. But I prefer organic coconut oil myself because of the other nutrients that are in it. There are a lot of vitamins and minerals and other things in coconut oil. If it's refined, they may be removed.

Some people can't stand the fragrance of coconut. I don't understand that, but...

PEGGY: I think it's... But, okay.

DR NEWPORT: But for people that don't like the smell of coconut, there is refined coconut oil, and it even comes as organic coconut oil.

PEGGY: Oh, even though it's refined.

DR NEWPORT: Yeah, even though it's refined. You can find organic, refined coconut oil.

PEGGY: And these are not expensive.

DR NEWPORT: These are not expensive. This is $10 at Sam's or Costco.

PEGGY: Costco has refined, organic coconut oil.

DR NEWPORT: Right. Right.

PEGGY: Nice, big jars.

DR NEWPORT: $10, and the other one was about $16 or $17, it usually runs. And you know, if you don't like the fragrance of coconut, you can use refined coconut oil, and you can cook with it.

PEGGY: You're going to cook your eggs in it? You're going to add it to your...? What are you going to do with this coconut oil?

DR NEWPORT: You can cook eggs. Yeah, yeah, you can do so many things with it. Just think of what you would do with butter, for example, or olive oil. Just different things that you would do with that. With straight coconut oil, I usually cook with it. You can cook eggs, scrambled eggs just soak it right up. I make frittatas with it. I cook vegetables in it.

PEGGY: Do you think you can spray it on your toast, or...?

DR NEWPORT: Yeah, yeah. I do stir fries with it. If you do a stir fry and use higher heat, you can actually add another – a little bit of another oil.

PEGGY: Like an olive oil?

DR NEWPORT: Like olive oil, or sesame oil, or peanut oil... Just a little bit of another oil will allow you to cook at a higher temperature.

PEGGY: I see. So the coconut oil, we want to keep at a lower temperature in order to maintain its properties.

DR NEWPORT: Yeah, medium temperature or below on the stove. In the oven, if you're putting it on something, 350° or below. The smoke point is at 350°, so it will start to smoke, and then it ruins the fat.

PEGGY: Okay, so we're beginning, we're building everything upon our delicious coconut oil, or our refined coconut oil, which has no flavor. And now what other products can we try – suppose you like chocolate?

DR NEWPORT: Okay, so if you like chocolate, this is a combination, roughly half dark chocolate and half coconut oil, and a little bit of honey – just enough to sweeten it. And this, you can make candies from it. This is a little candy cup, and you can put nuts, grated coconut, flaked coconut, a cherry... anything you can think of, or just plain chocolate, if you're a choco-holic.

You put it on a platter. You fill up the little cups, and you put it in the refrigerator, and an hour or so later it's solid.

PEGGY: You've got a delicious, healthy chocolate candy.

DR NEWPORT: A nice little dessert.

PEGGY: What else – okay. Coconut water has become, like, "the thing" these days.

DR NEWPORT: Yeah.

PEGGY: Does that also raise your ketone levels?

DR NEWPORT: No. Coconut water does not raise your ketone levels. A lot of people ask me about that. It has a lot of nutrients in it, though. It's got a good amount of potassium, a little bit of sodium. It's very hydrating. It was used as an IV fluid in Asia during World War II, and even some of the Americans used it if they ran out of straight IV fluid. It's similar to human plasma.

PEGGY: Oh, and it tastes good.

DR NEWPORT: Yes.

PEGGY: So it's not going to raise your ketone levels, but it is going to bring you some of the other benefits.

DR NEWPORT: This will not, no.

PEGGY: There are many benefits to the coconut.

DR NEWPORT: Yeah. The coconut is amazing, but one of the things I do with coconut water is I use coconut milk, which is mostly coconut oil, and I dilute it. I use it in smoothies. I drink it straight. I love coconut milk. And if you dilute a can of coconut milk with a can to a can-and-a-half of tap water or coconut water...

PEGGY: And then you can make it chocolate with a little bit of...

DR NEWPORT: You could make it chocolate.

PEGGY: Yeah.

DR NEWPORT: Five ounces of it would be equal to a tablespoon of coconut oil, if you dilute it with a can-and-a-half of water or coconut water.

PEGGY: So coconut milk, coconut, which we can put in our cereal, or...

DR NEWPORT: Yes, you can put it on cereal. You can drink it straight. It's delicious.

PEGGY: Just drink it straight, okay. Coconut water, coconut milk, coconut oil... What else do we have there? We have... Well, maybe we should talk about MCT oil, actually.

DR NEWPORT: Oh, yeah.

PEGGY: Because that is part of how you work to keep the ketone levels up.

DR NEWPORT: Prepared for Steve, right. There are many different brands. This is one of the least expensive, just as good as the others, in my opinion. This is about $17 a quart online, $17 or $18 on Amazon.

PEGGY: Turn it toward – so we can see. It's MCT.

DR NEWPORT: MCT.

PEGGY: Medium chain triglyceride oil.

DR NEWPORT: Medium chain triglyceride oil.

PEGGY: Okay.

DR NEWPORT: So this is extracted from coconut oil, and coconut oil is about 60% medium chain triglycerides. It will raise ketone levels higher. MCT oil is the basis of the medical food. One of the medium chain triglycerides is what's used in the medical food Axona.

PEGGY: A-X-O-N-A.

DR NEWPORT: Which is where I got the idea to use coconut oil and MCT oil with my husband. It's a prescription medical food. And it's available over the counter as coconut oil or MCT oil, so yes. You don't necessarily have to get a prescription to do this.

PEGGY: So you don't necessarily need a prescription anyway if all you're experiencing is just a little bit of those symptoms, "Mmm... Not quite as sharp as I use to be..." So you can take some of the MCT oil, mix it...

DR NEWPORT: In almost anything.

PEGGY: We can add it into our delicious coconut milk.

DR NEWPORT: Right. You can put it in the coconut milk smoothies. You could use it as part of salad dressing. I use it a lot that way. I'll put two or three teaspoons on my salad, and then two or three teaspoons of another salad dressing.

PEGGY: But on a practical level, I would cook with coconut oil. I'm not sure I would cook with MCT oil.

DR NEWPORT: This smokes at 320°, quite a bit lower. It tends to foam a little bit, too, when you cook with it.

PEGGY: So it might not be the best for cooking.

DR NEWPORT: Not the best for cooking.

PEGGY: But you could add it to a food afterwards.

DR NEWPORT: Right.

PEGGY: And make your veggies, and just put them on...

DR NEWPORT: Almost anything. Soup... You could put it in tea or coffee. It floats to the top a little bit. There's a company, many companies, several of them, now, that make a powdered MCT oil. This one happens to be from Japan. So when you add this to coffee, it's like adding creamer to your coffee.

PEGGY: Oh.

DR NEWPORT: But it's a great way to get MCT oil in.

PEGGY: Now, on a practical level, if you're travelling...

DR NEWPORT: Travelling.

PEGGY: And you want to take your packets.

DR NEWPORT: You take your packets. It could go in your carry on.

PEGGY: I mean, you wouldn't want to pack that big jar – yeah.

DR NEWPORT: You wouldn't want to pack this.

PEGGY: You don't want to pack that.

DR NEWPORT: Then there's a little tiny bottle... I have a three-ounce bottle of MCT oil, which is probably a sample bottle from a company, but you could carry a little bottle like that. Three ounces – now they allow up to three ounces of liquids in your carry on.

So if you like using straight MCT oil, you could just carry a little bottle of it.

PEGGY: Excellent! Okay, what about baking?

DR NEWPORT: Let's see... There is coconut flour... and... here it is.

PEGGY: It's right back there. Coconut flour.

DR NEWPORT: They have recipes on here. This is gluten free, so people that are trying to avoid gluten can use coconut flour, and again, it's fat. It's got carbohydrate in it, but most of the carbohydrate is fiber. It's not sugar. Just a little bit of sugar.

PEGGY: You raised the subject of gluten, and many people, although they might not show up as celiac disease, or whatever, do have a sensitivity to gluten that could influence their cognitive powers.

DR NEWPORT: Their brain, right.

PEGGY: It might be dulling them, so if they want to cut back, still have sweets, cut back on the gluten, there's coconut flour to nourish the brain instead of to dull the brain.

DR NEWPORT: Right. And one of the fun things I like to do with this is to make chicken tenders, or fish fingers, to coat it in coconut flour, along with – I usually put a little parmesan, a little salt and pepper... roll it in that, and cook it in coconut oil.

PEGGY: Invite me to dinner. It sounds great!

DR NEWPORT: It's delicious. It's very good.

PEGGY: It sounds great. Okay, so we've got a whole lot of products here that probably we're not aware of. What about coconut sugar?

DR NEWPORT: Yes, coconut sugar. It does not have coconut oil in it, so it will not raise your ketones.

PEGGY: Okay, but it's got the other stuff?

DR NEWPORT: But it is a natural sugar that's –

PEGGY: It's got the minerals, and the other nutrients...?

DR NEWPORT: It's got the vitamins and minerals and other things. I've even seen this in packets in Panera now, for your coffee or tea.

PEGGY: So again, going more mainstream.

DR NEWPORT: It's a refined sugar, so this is an unrefined sugar, basically.

PEGGY: So if you must have sugar, this is a better way to go.

DR NEWPORT: This may be a better way.

PEGGY: It's not going to spike your blood sugar... not as much as refined sugar.

Suppose somebody's watching this, and they are looking to get sharper. They're looking to get some of that speed and focus and alertness back, and they want to incorporate ketones. They want to raise ketone levels. How do they go – How do you start? Is it something you can just jump into, or do you...? How do you recommend starting a program like this?

DR NEWPORT: Well, some people are lucky, like my husband, and they can take two tablespoons of coconut oil right away, and they don't have a problem. But many people do have a problem. They can have an upset stomach, diarrhea, indigestion... if you try to take too much too fast.

So I normally recommend to people, if they're starting with coconut oil, to start with perhaps one teaspoon, two or three times a day with food.

PEGGY: So start by incorporating it into the food.

DR NEWPORT: Into the food.

PEGGY: Not by itself.

DR NEWPORT: Right. And with MCT oil, probably it's a little more potent, as far as possibly causing diarrhea. So using maybe a half teaspoon for starters, two or three times a day, with food. If you take it with food you're much less likely to have a problem like that. MCT oil's tasteless, so it disappears into the food. You can put it in almost anything. You could take it straight, but just eat at the same time.

PEGGY: Just eat, okay. So that's important if you want to avoid indigestion or other associated problems, you incorporate it into your diet with food.

DR NEWPORT: With food into your meals.

PEGGY: And what are we aiming for? If we're seeking to raise ketone levels consistently throughout the day in order to keep our brain fully functioning, as long as we're awake, what's our goal here? How many teaspoons or tablespoons per day?

DR NEWPORT: If you have a little bit of a problem, or you're looking at it for prevention, I suggest trying to get up somewhere from three to five tablespoons a day.

PEGGY: Tablespoons, not teaspoons. Tablespoons.

DR NEWPORT: Right. With somebody with a disease like Alzheimer's, aiming more for four to six tablespoons or more if the person can handle it, and just increasing very gradually with that in mind.

One interesting thing that people might like to hear is there's a doctor in Canada– he's a PhD.

He has looked at the brains of people with mild to moderate Alzheimer's disease, mainly mild Alzheimer's, and normal, elderly adults. He does glucose and ketone PET scans, and he has found the areas of the brain that are affected by Alzheimer's that do not take up glucose normally do take up ketones normally. It implies that the cells are still there. They're like cars without gas in them.

PEGGY: Right, so...

DR NEWPORT: So they're waiting for a fuel.

PEGGY: They need to be tanked, and then you're good to go.

DR NEWPORT: So if you can provide ketones as an alternative fuel, those cells could function better.

PEGGY: That's very important to know, that there's a possibility of revival of damaged brain cells by fueling them through ketones.

So we're aiming at the ranges of three to five tablespoons for people who are still functioning, but...

DR NEWPORT: Maybe a little problem.

PEGGY: Beginnings of problems.

DR NEWPORT: Or they don't have a problem yet, but they're worried that they might develop a problem.

PEGGY: They worry that perhaps it runs in their family, and as you point out, people can begin to develop Alzheimer's decades before first symptoms, as we know now from brain scans.

DR NEWPORT: Decades.

PEGGY: So if it runs in your family, this is something that you can be doing to have a consistent level of nourishment in the brain and prevent future problems. So that's three to five for prevention, and just the beginnings of problems, and four to six tablespoons...

DR NEWPORT: Or more.

PEGGY: ...or more.

DR NEWPORT: If you can handle it.

PEGGY: If your digestive system can handle it, even more for people dealing with actual dementia situations.

DR NEWPORT: Right.

PEGGY: Okay. Are there other benefits... You're going to see increased brain sharpness. Are there other benefits that you might see from taking coconut oil – from raising ketone levels?

DR NEWPORT: Some people have physical endurance, even. They actually did a study at the Byrd Alzheimer's Institute. It was in mice, but they were looking at the effects of raising ketones in normal mice, and in mice that were an Alzheimer's model. And one of the things they found was that there was marked increase in endurance, both for the normal mice and for the Alzheimer's mice. They basically ran on a little treadmill until they fell off.

PEGGY: So it's a sports fuel.

DR NEWPORT: Yes, and it doubled the amount of time they were able to spend on the treadmill.

PEGGY: That's kind of amazing.

DR NEWPORT: Isn't that interesting?

PEGGY: Now, MCT oil is used by athletes, is that correct?

DR NEWPORT: It's used by body builders.

PEGGY: By body builders.

DR NEWPORT: To increase their lean body mass.

PEGGY: Lean body mass.

DR NEWPORT: Right.

PEGGY: We want to shed the fat, and we want to gain the muscle. And MCT oil can help promote that.

DR NEWPORT: Right. In Japan, the company that's making these products now for Alzheimer's, for 20 years they've been studying MCT oil, making it and studying it for weight loss and prevention of weight gain. They're allowed to say in Japan that this could prevent gaining fat, because MCT's are not stored as fat. They're burned immediately as energy.

PEGGY: So they don't get stored as fat. I'm glad we're on the topic of fat, gaining fat, gaining weight... All that we've been discussing is oils. We've been discussing saturated fats, and we've all kind of been programmed to go, "Oh, no, no, no." Saturated fats that may cause our doctors to say, "What are you doing with these saturated fats?" So how do we understand that?

DR NEWPORT: MCT's – medium chain triglycerides – are all saturated fats. But it's the longer chain saturated fats that are the ones we've actually studied that may be of concern, possibly. There are more and more studies now showing that saturated fat isn't nearly the problem that it was thought to be.

Same with high cholesterol, elevated cholesterol might not be quite the problem it was thought to be. However, these are medium chain triglycerides. They're converted either to ketones or burned immediately as energy. They're not stored as fat.

PEGGY: They're burned as energy immediately. This is a crucial point. You're not going to get fat from these, because they're going to convert into energy, which you will probably feel very fast. Isn't that correct? I mean, if you feel more energy...

DR NEWPORT: Yeah, if you're someone that's going to respond to it, you'll probably notice it right away.

PEGGY: As your mice on the treadmills did. You're going to have more physical and mental endurance. Okay, so is that what we're going to tell our cardiologist?

DR NEWPORT: We're going to talk to him about it. I suggest getting the doctor involved, especially if you do have health issues, in particular, cardiac issues... Studies really still need to be done with all of this. But the doctor could follow your lipid panel. You could incorporate it very slowly. You might tend more towards MCT oil than coconut oil, because MCTs are really the fats we're trying to get. And you know, following the lipid level over time could tell you, is this a problem for you or not? So if you can enlist the help of your doctor in this, that would be helpful.

PEGGY: Yes, you want your doctor working with you, for sure. Let's talk about coconut oil and these other products that we looked at – MCT oil – as part of an overall, brain-healthy diet.

You've written two books, so let's take a look at your first book, which really raised a tremendous amount of awareness about coconut oil and its beneficial effects on Alzheimer's. The title was *Alzheimer's Disease: What if There Was a Cure?* The story of ketones.

DR NEWPORT: Yes, I wrote this book, really, to try to get the message out about coconut oil. I had written an article about two months after Steve responded, and that was after many letters written to politicians and media people, trying to bring attention to the idea of using ketones as an alternative fuel.

The medical food was still a year away from coming out, and I felt that it needed urgent attention, this whole idea, because of how many millions of people are dealing with Alzheimer's – about 5.2 million in this country, and 35 million worldwide, and it's growing. It's expected to triple by 2050.

PEGGY: And it's happening younger, as...

DR NEWPORT: Younger and younger, like my husband.

PEGGY: Younger people, as more and more people get diabetes, which is associated with Alzheimer's.

DR NEWPORT: Right. You're at a much higher risk of developing dementia if you have diabetes. So I wanted to get the message out about it, and basically the first part of the book talks about our story – Steve's decline into Alzheimer's, and then coming up out of the abyss with the coconut oil... and then trying to get the message out.

I have a lot of caregiver reports – people who emailed me with results, improvements. Not everybody improves, but there were many people who did, some dramatically, some more gradually. I include a lot of those in here.

The science of ketones – what are the fundamentals? I try to word it in such a way that the average layperson can understand it, but doctors are not insulted by it. And I have doctors read it, and they were very happy with how much information they got about Alzheimer's out of this.

PEGGY: You know, you raise a crucial point, which is that you're kind of the point person out there in the public eye about coconut oil and its effects on the brain. So you've heard from literally hundreds of people.

DR NEWPORT: Right.

PEGGY: This isn't now just you and your particular circumstance. This is –

DR NEWPORT: Right. At that point, it was the very beginning. It was a case of one.

PEGGY: Right. And now you've heard from... How many people have you heard from?

DR NEWPORT: As of a couple of years ago it was over 400 that had had improvement, and it's many more now. I just stopped counting.

PEGGY: Too many to count.

DR NEWPORT: Too many to count, yeah.

PEGGY: So you've reached the point where you've helped so many people you can't even count how many people, and people are reporting improved brain function.

DR NEWPORT: Right, right. Improved memory and cognition, improved social interaction, improved mood... Some people say their depression lifted, which is what happened with my husband. He started saying he felt like he had a future again.

PEGGY: What about a common complaint that people have as they get a little bit older: It's just the word recall, the tip of the tongue-itis.

DR NEWPORT: Right.

PEGGY: Is this going to help with that?

DR NEWPORT: It could, it could help with finishing sentences, being able to finish your thoughts and your ideas, and making conversation with other people, carrying on a conversation. It's often elusive in Alzheimer's disease. You can be on a different wavelength.

PEGGY: And of course, people with Alzheimer's have sleep disturbances.

DR NEWPORT: They have sleep disturbances. Some people have reported improved sleep. For some people, if they take MCT oil before they go to sleep they have vivid dreams. I've heard that a lot.

PEGGY: Oh! Could be a good thing.

DR NEWPORT: Yeah.

PEGGY: Might that not help so many people who have sleep problems, especially as they get older? Might keeping your body, your ketone levels consistent throughout the day, might that help with sleep?

DR NEWPORT: Just overall it can help your brain function better, and that's one thing personally I notice. I take MCT's before I go to sleep. I feel like I sleep better.

PEGGY: That's key.

DR NEWPORT: And I remember my dreams. Steve couldn't remember dreams for years. And one of the things that happened fairly early on is he started remembering dreams.

PEGGY: Yeah.

DR NEWPORT: And for somebody with Alzheimer's to remember something like a dream was rather amazing.

PEGGY: That is rather amazing. Okay, so now your new book is...

DR NEWPORT: My new book is *The Coconut Oil and Low Carb Solution for Alzheimer's, Parkinson's, and Other Diseases*. And I wish it had diabetes in the list here, too. The book is really relevant for people with diabetes, but...

This book is a little bit more practical. It's a companion to the other book, but it goes into more detail about how to use coconut oil in the diet, fairly quickly in the book.

And also reducing the carbohydrate, especially the added sugar in the diet. That's become a very big problem in the last few decades of this last century – added sugar has been greatly on the increase. In conjunction with a low fat diet, somehow you have to make up those calories, and what is it going to be? It's going to be carbohydrate, usually. So there are a lot of added sugars in foods now.

Basically, this book teaches people how to reduce carbohydrates in their diet. Very practical, reasonable... It's not like a very strict induction Atkin's Diet, you know, where you're completely deprived of carbohydrate. But really, teaching people how to exercise portion control, and still maybe use one slice of bread instead of two slices of bread, a half a cup of rice instead of a whole cup of rice, whole grain rice or something. But just ways of cutting out excessive sugar in the diet through choosing foods wisely.

And what happens is that if you can get below 60 grams of carbs a day or so in your diet, you can actually raise ketone levels a little bit, and then you can further build on that and get higher levels by using coconut and MCT oil along with it. We've measured MCT oil – or, ketone levels after doing this, and adding the effects of a low carb diet will further increase ketone levels.

Dr. Cunnane, whom I mentioned in another section, is a PhD in Canada who's looking at glucose and ketone PET scans, and he has found that the higher your plasma level of ketones, the greater the percentage of energy you can provide to the brain. So he feels that using MCT oil in the diet can potentially provide prevention.

PEGGY: So we want to eat a brain-healthy diet. In the overall diet we want to keep our ketone levels consistently high throughout the day by using some of the products you've shown us here, certainly coconut oil. And we want to reduce our carbs, and thereby, also raise our ketones.

DR NEWPORT: Right.

PEGGY: So that's the overall brain-healthy plan.

DR NEWPORT: Right.

PEGGY: And is there anybody who shouldn't do this?

DR NEWPORT: People who are allergic to coconut might have a problem, although MCT oil might be okay for those people. I mean, that's a possibility. Depending on how severe their allergy is, they might be able to experiment a little bit with that.

PEGGY: Most people aren't allergic to coconut oil.

DR NEWPORT: Most people are not. Very few people are... it's pretty rare. People with liver failure should use these oils cautiously or not at all. The medium chain triglycerides are metabolized in the liver, and fat in general is not good for somebody who's in liver failure. And for people with very rare enzyme defects, a couple of very rare enzyme defects, MCTs would not be appropriate.

PEGGY: But other than those conditions – which are relatively rare – unless you're allergic to coconuts, or you're in late-stage liver failure, or with a very special enzyme condition, this is a great way to regularly eat for your brain, for brain health.

DR NEWPORT: Right, right. And if you have a serious cardiac problem or other chronic illness, it would be a good idea to get your doctor involved in this. And perhaps monitor the lipid levels.

PEGGY: Right. One other thing I want to mention is that this is good for other conditions. For instance, what are some of the other conditions that eating a low carb diet and using coconuts can improve?

DR NEWPORT: There are many of them, diabetes being number one, I would say, just because of the sheer number of people who are dealing with diabetes. If you're 75 or older you have a high risk – three quarters of that population will have either diabetes or pre-diabetes.

PEGGY: That's stunning.

DR NEWPORT: It's a very high percentage of the population.

PEGGY: 75% of people over 75.

DR NEWPORT: Right. And this is a relatively new phenomenon that's been growing. It's really gone to epidemic proportions, along with Alzheimer's and some of these other diseases that have been on the rise. Parkinson's disease responds, ALS – Lou Gehrig disease – multiple sclerosis...

PEGGY: Really?

DR NEWPORT: Yeah. Dr. Terry Wahls is a physician who is an internist. She was a traditional physician, and she found that by getting your vitamins from natural foods – from vegetables of different colors, and different types of vegetables – she had great benefit from that, and she's written a book called *The Wahls Protocol*. Now she has The Wahls Protocol Plus, which includes coconut oil.

PEGGY: There you go.

DR NEWPORT: She has found additional benefit to people with MS from using coconut oil.

PEGGY: So we're looking at the spectrum of neurodegenerative diseases.

DR NEWPORT: Right.

PEGGY: That all seem to respond. Here's another problem people have as they get older: aches and pains.

DR NEWPORT: Right. Yeah, that is a good question. That's where reducing sugar can come in.

PEGGY: In terms of the inflammation.

DR NEWPORT: Right, right. But added sugar is...

PEGGY: What about coconut oil as a massage oil...?

DR NEWPORT: Yeah, as a massage oil, yes. Coconut oil is absorbed, and it can be absorbed by the muscles. The medium chains are used directly by the muscles. People with ALS – they're a group locally – they call it the "Deanna Protocol" for Deanna, who has improved. I mean, she drastically slowed down the progress of that disease. Most people are gone in three to five years after they develop ALS – that is, Lou Gehrig disease.

PEGGY: Yes.

DR NEWPORT: And they ingest coconut oil, a number of other supplements, but they also massage coconut oil, and they find benefit from that. They have problems with cramping and muscle wasting, symptoms they have with that disease, and they feel that they get benefit from massaging coconut oil.

PEGGY: Coconut oil is supposed to be good for the skin, too.

DR NEWPORT: Yes. People use it in their hair. They put it in their hair and put a cap on their head overnight, and then wash it out in the morning. It's a great moisturizer.

PEGGY: Very, very miraculous. The coconut oil miracle!

Basically, this is good for almost everybody who is interested in nourishing their brain for the long haul – and there's short-term benefit as well.

DR NEWPORT: Right.

PEGGY: So thank you so much, Dr. Newport, for sharing with us your knowledge and your practical expertise in how to incorporate ketones into our daily diet. And thank you for watching. I hope you learned some useful tips, some products that can be part of your daily routine and raise the ketone levels in your body to keep your brain nourished to prevent Alzheimer's, and to just boost your brain every day for higher function. Thank you.

Interview with Joseph Maroon, M.D.

PEGGY SARLIN: Hello, I'm Peggy Sarlin, and today I'm in Pittsburgh, Pennsylvania, where I'm so excited to speak with Dr. Joseph Maroon, a world-renowned neurosurgeon. Dr. Maroon is the first surgeon I've spoken to in the series, so he brings us a whole new perspective on brain health.

Dr. Maroon is the Medical Director of World Wrestling Entertainment and also of the Pittsburgh Steelers, so he certainly knows about head trauma and brain injury, and how to heal them, and that's important stuff.

Dr. Maroon is an Ironman athlete. He is an expert in nutrition, which is not typical of surgeons, and he has deep insight into burnout, extreme stress, because he's lived it. I think you're going to get so much practical wisdom from what Dr. Maroon has to say. So welcome, Dr. Maroon.

DR MAROON: Thank you so much, Peggy. I'm very much looking forward to our conversation, and bringing these messages to your audience.

PEGGY: So Doctor, I think a lot of people who are watching us may be caregivers to people with Alzheimer's or some other serious problem. And we have talked a lot in the series about what goes on in the brain of people with dementia. But what we haven't talked about is what goes on in the brain of their caregiver – of somebody who's living with relentless stress, day after day – and they need help, too. So tell us about the caregivers and their stress load.

DR MAROON: Peggy, it's an absolutely huge problem, when you think about the number of patients with dementia, with traumatic brain injuries, with families of kids who have opioid problems, of single mothers and – wherever they live, and, as you said, the overwhelming, intense stress.

So we have to ask ourselves, what does stress do to the body and to the brain? We know these people feel overwhelmed, overworked, overcommitted, and, clearly, overstressed. And when that happens, the body, in its protective mode, releases a hormone called cortisol, which is initially protective, but when elevated in a chronic way, has very negative effects on the body and also the brain. In fact, it literally destroys brain cells, particularly in that area of the brain that subserves memory.

So people say, "I can't remember this. I can't remember that" when they're under chronic stress, and it's because they're actually damaging their brain as well as their blood vessels, their heart, and other parts of the body.

PEGGY: So cortisol is kind of a key figure in this drama that we're going to discuss, the drama of stress, and it's something that we need. It's a hormone, it's a neurotransmitter?

DR MAROON: It's a hormone...

PEGGY: It's a hormone.

DR MAROON: ...that's protective to the body. It's part of the "fight or flight" mechanism that evolutionarily, we've been imbued with for hundreds of thousands of years.

It's cortisol, and it's also adrenaline, or epinephrine that enable us to avoid danger, to get out of difficult situations quickly. But when the danger's over, we go back to a normal homeostatic way, you might say. But when it's chronically elevated, as you said, in the caregivers or individuals who are caring for a spouse who is becoming progressively more incapacitated, what happens is this hormone continues to be elevated, as do other hormones.

This contributes to depression, to futility, to feeling overwhelmed, and then to a downward spiral that really is hard to stop unless we do very specific things that I discuss in my book, *Square One: A Simple Guide to a Balanced Life,* in which I outline the measures that can be taken by anyone in extreme stress conditions to, hopefully, reverse the process.

PEGGY: Well, you're telling us something very important – and very scary, which is that if we're under extreme stress for a long period of time, our brain is continually besieged by cortisol, and cortisol is continuously killing the brain cells. Our brains are being murdered.

DR MAROON: Overstimulation will result in the death of brain cells, particularly in an area of the brain, in the temporal area here, an area called the "hippocampus," which subserves memory.

PEGGY: And many of the people in our audience, who are interested in Alzheimer's, know that the hippocampus is where Alzheimer's begins.

DR MAROON: Precisely. The first thing that happens is the "I can't remember my keys. I can't remember going to the store." And then emotional disorders also subsequently come, where there are significant mood changes, impulsivity, anger, difficulty to control emotions and activities. And all of this, obviously, is a function of dysfunctional brain workings.

PEGGY: So we have this kind of horrible irony going on, where you may be a caregiver to somebody with Alzheimer's, and the stress of that situation is flooding your brain with cortisol, which is precisely attacking the hippocampus, the area that is setting you up to potentially get Alzheimer's.

DR MAROON: Precisely. That's exactly what happens in the story. So those who are committed to helping their spouse, their child, their loved one – unless it's in a way where they are aware of the over-commitment that it sometimes requires, and take very specific steps to obviate that stress – it can really become even more disruptive.

PEGGY: Well, we're going to talk about how to obviate that stress, as you say. But first, let's also just look at some other professions or situations... You've mentioned caring for a child. What are some other people at risk – you and I have spoken about the fact that doctors are prone to extreme stress.

DR MAROON: This is a horrible problem in physicians.

Recently, the Mayo Clinic published a study in which they looked at several thousand physicians, and concluded that, several years ago, the incidence of burnout was 30 or 40%. It's now up to 49%, and in my profession, neurosurgery, it's 57%.

PEGGY: A majority of...

DR MAROON: So the majority of neurosurgeons are under significant stress, to the point where they have one of the main determinations of burnout: Number one, it's "overwhelm," exhaustion, mental exhaustion, where they feel they simply have a difficult time coping.

The second is depersonalization, meaning they lose contact emotionally with their family, their colleagues, even their patients. They may become irritable, cynical, sarcastic. It's a symptom of the depersonalization.

And the other symptom of burnout, the third, is they don't feel fulfilled in their profession, in their work. What's it all about, Alfie? Why am I doing this? I'm killing myself for this. So 50% of physicians have one of these symptoms now.

And the other problem in caregivers, as well as physicians, and nurses, and other healthcare providers, is that of suicide, suicide ideation. Four hundred physicians committed suicide last year.

PEGGY: Oh, that's horrible.

DR MAROON: And among medical students... there was a recent paper in the *Journal of the American Medical Association* where they looked at burnout in medical students. And seven to ten percent of medical students at some point have suicidal ideation. In other words, it enters their mind, and it's a consideration. So the consequences of not dealing with this in a proper way are horrendous.

PEGGY: You differentiated stress from burnout. There's stress, and I think we all know about it, we've all – everybody's – experienced stress. But when it sustains over a period of time, it can devolve into burnout, and the way you described it, that seemed to entail personality change. Is that the key factor...?

DR MAROON: Well, I think you're touching on an incredibly important point. There's good stress, and there's bad stress. Distress – D-I-S – and eustress – E-U stress. And if you draw a chart, and you have a parabolic curve, where the curtain goes up, and it gets to a point, and then it goes down, and you have good stress on this side, and once you get over a threshold, it's bad stress, it's...

As you mentioned, I do triathlons, and I've been doing these for many years. And any athlete knows that unless you stress your body, you don't get better. You don't get stronger. You don't get faster.

PEGGY: Right.

DR MAROON: So stress is good. Stress is very good – as long as it's controlled. When it gets into distress, in other words, when it becomes overwhelming, then it takes a very serious toll, depending on the severity of the stress.

PEGGY: Well, I think one thing that differentiates stress from burnout is when you are constantly in a position that is out of your control. So let's go back to the caregiver.

DR MAROON: Yes.

PEGGY: Crisis after crisis after crisis, for which you may not have the resources, the energy, the time, the money, the knowledge... And things are happening that you can't control, and that is extraordinarily dangerous, I suppose, long-term, to be carrying that kind of a load.

DR MAROON: It's very dangerous, and unfortunately, it's epidemic in our society and in our country today. When you go into the various areas of Pittsburgh, and you see that 60-70% of the children are born out of wedlock to single mothers... so it begins very early, in terms of...

PEGGY: So the stress of the mother...

DR MAROON: ...how the stress of the mother actually gets conveyed *in utero* – in the womb – to the brain of the child. We know that we have a terrible situation with crack babies born in Magee-Womens Hospital, here at the University of Pittsburgh. And their mothers who abuse their bodies during pregnancy with cocaine, with various types of drugs, even with marijuana, can have deleterious long-term effects on the baby, on the baby's brains, inclinations, synaptic connections, and the neuroplasticity, or growth of the baby's brain. These kids come out of the womb in withdrawal.

It starts very early in terms of... we talked about resilience, you know. We both have been very fortunate in our lives to have gone through cataclysmic types of stresses, and somehow we've been able to survive that, and come out the other side better off.

And again, that's the story I tell in my book, *Square One* – that there are ways of coping with stress that are very healthy, without drugs, without pharmaceutical drugs.

PEGGY: Right, right.

DR MAROON: Without pharmaceutical drugs.

PEGGY: Right. So let's start giving help to people who are watching this and who are coping with stress. We're going to get into your book, which is a whole philosophy. But before we get into something more elaborate, let's start with something simple. After people watch this, they then go to the store and buy some supplements that are going to help them fortify their body and build their resilience in a time of extreme stress?

DR MAROON: Well, supplements are one part of the whole picture...

PEGGY: Yes.

DR MAROON: ...as you well know.

PEGGY: Yes.

DR MAROON: And we talk about epigenetics, or the epigenetic factors, those factors that tell our genes whether to make good proteins or bad proteins, to promote inflammation in our body, or anti-inflammation. If we eat an inappropriate diet with a lot of sugar and soft drinks, and trans-fatty acids on our French fries, and hormone-infused beef, it's going to tell our genes to make inflammatory agents, and inflammation is the common genesis of Alzheimer's, of stroke, of myocardial infarction, or heart attacks, and damage to our joints and endothelium.

If we eat a Mediterranean diet, take the right supplements that I will get to, exercise, control our environmental toxins, avoid too much alcohol, avoid smoking, and control stress, our bodies make anti-inflammatory agents that lead to a healthy heart, a healthy brain, and healthy joints.

So the supplements, yes, there are certain supplements that I take every day. The first is Omega-3 fatty acids, fish oil. I take a product, Omax3, that is a very high concentration of EPA, eicosapentaenoic acid versus DHA, which has a very high anti-inflammatory component, because I work out a lot and I stress my body a lot.

I take another product called nicotinamide riboside made by a company, ChromaDex, and this product is essential for mitochondrial support. One of the leading theories of aging, why we look and get older, and why we develop the various diseases that you're focusing upon in this session is because of the malfunction of mitochondria.

Mitochondria are little organelles in each cell of our body that convert glucose, or sugar, and oxygen into ATP. ATP is the energy molecule that drives everything we do, every cell in terms of its energy. Nicotinamide riboside helps in making NAD, which is a precursor of ATP. NAD is essential in the making in our cells of ATP.

So I take this every day, and I feel it helps with energy. It helps with metabolism of fat, trans fatty acids, our fat in our liver, and it's also neuroprotective. Vitamin D3, I think, is an essential item in terms of neuro-protection, as well as endothelial protection. The endothelium is a lining of our blood vessels. We need to take care of the lining of our blood vessels, because it leads to heart disease and also strokes.

PEGGY: Right.

DR MAROON: So vitamin D3 is an essential vitamin, and also magnesium is involved in 300 different chemical reactions in our body. And particularly if you work out hard or sweat a lot, magnesium gets depleted, and it's essential for, again, cellular support.

So these are some of the things that I think are really important to add when you're under stress. Another is resveratrol. Resveratrol is a natural product found in red wine and also in grapes. I don't want you to take too much red wine, but one glass for women, two glasses for men are thought to have significant healthy benefits, just like dark chocolate. So you can drink a little wine, and eat a little dark chocolate...

PEGGY: That sounds good.

DR MAROON: ...and help yourself.

PEGGY: I'm less stressed already, just thinking about it.

DR MAROON: You're helping yourself. But it's another antioxidant, neuroprotective agent that is in the supplement range that I think that is important, as well as probiotics. In terms of our microbiome, the health of our gut is a reflection of about 70% of the immunity that we develop – it comes from our intestinal tract and the bacteria in our gut. So gut health is extremely important to brain health. There's a clear-cut gut-brain reaction, as you well know.

PEGGY: Okay, so for people who are watching this, who are living very stressful lives right now, the first thing they've learned is that their brains are being affected by the stress. They've learned their brains are being affected directly on the hippocampus, and they're becoming vulnerable to that kind of decay, Alzheimer's, dementia. And their brains are probably getting inflamed as well.

So once they know this, they can understand, "I have to start taking action to protect myself. And something I can do that's simple – I can get up just like Dr. Maroon does. I can get up in the morning. I can take Omega-3." If they're vegetarians, and they don't want to take fish oil, can they take krill oil instead?

DR MAROON: Krill oil's a very good supplement, yes.

PEGGY: Okay, and they can also take... the one I can't remember, because it's a long, complicated...

DR MAROON: Nicotinamide riboside, NR.

PEGGY: NR is easier. I can remember NR.

DR MAROON: NR, and it's by ChromaDex, a company in California.

PEGGY: Okay, so we've got our fish oil, our NR, resveratrol, Vitamin D3... You may have mentioned...

DR MAROON: Probiotic.

PEGGY: Probiotic, to keep that healthy...

DR MAROON: Gut health.

PEGGY: ...gut-brain connection; magnesium, which you burn up during stress. So you're already given people something practical. You can go to the store, and you can start taking these today, and start feeling better.

DR MAROON: Well, I don't want to mislead our audience, Peggy, in the sense that it's not all in a pill. It's excellent. As I said, it's multifactorial. It's one of the things that's, I think, important to do, because our diets are not as healthy as they should be, generally, in the United States.

But the most important thing in caregivers that I've seen, patients who have had terrible problems – strokes and other things, brain tumors – is depression. It's the futility of not being able to do what they want to do to help the individual that leads to depression. So if you go to your doctor, what's the first thing the doctor gives you for depression?

PEGGY: An antidepressant.

DR MAROON: Precisely. And then, if you can't sleep, what does he give you?

PEGGY: A sleeping pill.

DR MAROON: Exactly. And if you're too anxious, what does he give you?

PEGGY: What's that, Xanax?

DR MAROON: Xanax. So what happens is you come home with three different prescriptions. Now let me rhetorically ask you, what is the most effective antidepressant, the most effective?

PEGGY: I happen to know.

DR MAROON: It's exercise.

PEGGY: Yes.

DR MAROON: It's physical aerobic activity. Studies have been done in patients who have been depressed. The researchers put one group on antidepressants and anxiolytics, and they put the other group in a structured exercise program, three to five times a week. The patients who have been on the exercise program invariably improve, and don't need the drugs.

Meaning, the first thing the caregiver can do is get out and walk around the block once, and then twice, and then three times, and try to get in 8,000 to 10,000 steps a day, as we talk about now with our FitBits, and our pedometers. But the reason – and you know the answer to this, but I'm going to ask the audience – why does exercise work as an antidepressant? Why? What's it do to the brain?

PEGGY: Tell us.

DR MAROON: It does several things. Number one, it increases a molecule in our brain called BDNF – brain-derived neurotrophic factor. Our brain releases this molecule, and it does three things. It actually creates new brain cells. So the brain cells that we lose from the stress, we can replace with exercise.

Number two, it increases the connections between brain cells that are called synapses. It increases the connections wherein memory is encoded, and it aids our memory, and also it enhances what's called neuroplasticity, the ability of the brain to regenerate, and to reheal itself, to make new tracks through the brains that are destroyed by stress.

So those are three things that just BDNF does. So when I get on my bike this afternoon, and I ride up the hill that we drove down to get here, I'm thinking, "Gosh, I'm getting my BDNF higher every time I stress myself."

But it does other things with the neurotransmitters, which are the chemicals between the connections of our brain. If your audience can follow this, let me just tell you a little bit about the complexity of the brain.

We have over 100 billion – billion – neurons, or transistors, or cells in our brain, our cortex. Cortex means outer layer. Each of those cells has up to thousands of connections. So the synapses, the connections, number in the trillions. When we interrupt these connections, malfunction occurs in different organ systems. We can enhance these.

Now, at each of the synaptic connections is a chemical that tells the next neuron what to do. These are called neurotransmitters. One of them is dopamine, the feel-good hormone that we also get from exercise, and that also gets released by narcotics, which is why you get addicted to them. These receptors crave more of the feeling good of dopamine. Serotonin, an antidepressant molecule, and also anandamide are neurotransmitters.

Very few people have heard about anandamide. Anandamide is the brain's own marijuana, if I might say. Why does marijuana give people euphoria, a high? It does it because there are receptors in the brain called the endocannabinoid. You've heard of cannabis? Endocannabinoid receptors.

PEGGY: Right.

DR MAROON: "Endo" meaning "within our own brain" – within us, endogenous. Marijuana gives us a high, a good feeling, because it attaches to these endocannabinoid receptors.

However, God, in his great glory, made us with our own endogenous – or inherent – marijuana. Anandamide is what it's called. It comes from the Indian Sanskrit word meaning bliss.

So when we exercise, and we get this good feeling, we're also releasing anandamide into our receptors. And you might imagine yourself maybe... No, I won't go there.

PEGGY: Oh, good.

DR MAROON: But anyway, this is all natural. And how do antidepressants work in the brain? They're now discovering that it's releasing BDNF.

PEGGY: Oh, really?

DR MAROON: Yeah, really.

PEGGY: Oh.

DR MAROON: So wouldn't you rather take a walk around the block, or up the hill, or through the woods, or take a swim in a lake, than take antidepressants that cost you thousands of dollars a year, have side effects, decrease your libido, and really are effective in maybe 50% of the people?

PEGGY: Well, what you're saying it's so profound because we're programmed to go to the doctor, get a pill. This makes me better. It's something extrinsic. It's something that we take from outside of ourselves to cure what's in us. And you're telling us that we're built to actually create all these positive biochemical interactions just through exercise.

DR MAROON: Peggy, think about 50,000 years ago, 100,000 years ago, when we were on the savanna in Africa and we had to survive stress every day. The saber-tooth tiger jumping out of the woods, or starvation and famine, feast and famine. Our bodies, to survive, have learned over hundreds of thousands of years how to handle stress.

We need to encourage it in today's modern day, kind of to reach back to those periods when we worked, even though we're not chasing and hunting our food, we need to get physical exercise, or do hard physical work.

And we also need to watch our diet. I mean, 60% of the people of the United States are obese or overweight.

PEGGY: 60%.

DR MAROON: The United States has the highest GDP in the world. Our length of survival, in terms of age – how many centenarians we have – we rank 31st.

PEGGY: Well, that's quite a discrepancy.

DR MAROON: So it doesn't matter how much money we're making, or the goods we're producing. Our lifestyle is deteriorating, in terms of what we put into our body as fuel.

Again, going back, I wasn't always a triathlete. And this is what I discuss in my book. I mean, I burned myself out in my early 40s. I was doing brain surgery one day, and the next week I literally had to quit my job, and I was working in a truck stop, filling up 18-wheelers and flipping burgers, because I burned out.

My life was all work. I lost my family. I lost my father. I ended up, for a year, dropping out of neurosurgery. I could not function. I was totally... I could do no more than fill up an 18-wheeler truck with diesel fuel.

So the thing is that it's not futile. I guess the message is, "Don't give up hope." There are ways, if we do it the right way, if we attend to our bodies, we attend to our minds with spirituality, meditation, prayer, if we reduce stress, and we eliminate the toxic factors in our diet, our air, our water as much as we can, there is hope for the caregiver. There is hope for those individuals who are burned out.

I've given several talks at different university hospitals. I'm speaking at Harvard next week, to the medical students there, about burnout. It's a terrible problem in the medical profession, from the medical student to the residents.

And we're initiating a program at the University of Pittsburgh in burnout – in wellness, actually. It's a wellness program that incorporates those four factors for the residents, so that they're aware of it. We're providing a gym for them. We're providing knowledge in healthy diet, and how to handle stress better, and also, how to avoid the things that will affect your immune system.

So it's multi-factorial, but there's hope. There are things that can be done, and I discuss this very extensively in my book.

PEGGY: So Dr. Maroon, you talked about your book, and I'd like to tell the audience about the book. This is Dr. Maroon's book, *Square One*. Excellent book, and you heard him mention his own story, that he went from being a neurosurgeon to working at a truck stop.

He tells that story here, and he tells how he overcame that through the philosophy of Square One, which we're about to go into, including the science behind it. So you can read in more detail about some of the science that Dr. Maroon is sharing with us today. I thought you would want to know about this book, *Square One*.

So okay, Doctor, Square One – you refer to the four sides of the square as your philosophy for overcoming stress. Let's go over the four sides.

DR MAROON: Absolutely. To go back just a bit, I was a very, very successful neurosurgeon at University Hospital, and then, because of overwork, because of stress, I ended up living in a farmhouse in the middle of winter, working in a very dilapidated truck stop that my father bequeathed to my mother. And I had to help her manage the family finances.

And so I'm wondering, what's a nice guy like this doing here? How did this happened to me? And

I realized for the first time, I had no insight into what I was doing that led me to this particular situation.

And I picked up a little book by William Danforth, who formed the Purina company back in the early 1900s, titled *I Dare You!* I'd received this in high school as an award, but I really never read it. And basically, he says, "I dare you to lead a balanced life." That got my attention, because I realized I was totally unbalanced.

And he said, "What I want you to do is to draw a square. On the top part of the square, put work. On this side of the square, put family/social. On the bottom side, spiritual, and on this side, physical." He said, "Now I want you to draw a square consistent with how much energy, time you put on each one of these sides."

So I sat down, and I drew my square, and it was an absolutely straight line, with no family, no spiritual, and absolutely no physical. I was 20 pounds overweight. And it was a flatline EKG, signifying death. It was all work.

PEGGY: Work, work, work.

DR MAROON: It was all work.

PEGGY: Brain surgeon.

DR MAROON: But I looked at that symbol, and I said... It didn't quite register. I saw I'm really out of balance.

And as luck, fortune, God would have it, I received a call from the banker who owned the mortgage on the truck stop, and he said, "Joe, let's go for a run. I think you need to get out." Run? I can't walk. I got short of breath climbing a flight of steps.

But I ended up going down to the Triadelphia, West Virginia high school track, and we made it around four times. I thought I would die. I said, "Never again." But that night I went home, and it was the first night I slept in four months.

PEGGY: Now, that's a key point. Let me just stop you there.

DR MAROON: The first night I slept.

PEGGY: Because stress makes it harder to sleep.

DR MAROON: Oh, my God.

PEGGY: And sleep is essential. So you've given us something very important: If we start exercising, even if we don't feel like it, and even if we're not doing that much, if it's more than were accustomed to, we're going to encourage our bodies to sleep.

DR MAROON: I tried sleeping pills. I tried melatonin. I tried natural remedies... everything to try to sleep.

PEGGY: Right.

DR MAROON: That was the first night I slept.

PEGGY: Key. Key point.

DR MAROON: So the next day, a lightbulb went off, and I said, "Gee, maybe it's related." So I went down to the same track by myself, and I did a mile and a half... then two miles... then three miles... And with each day, I felt my depression getting a little less, my ability to function improve. My brain was being rewired, literally.

PEGGY: Right.

DR MAROON: And then, about then, I also picked up a Bible that I had read very faithfully in high school and college, and I started getting back to the spiritual underpinnings that I really had lived by throughout my whole training, and in most of my medical career, but which had slipped away. And I also reconnected with my kids and my family.

So very slowly, each side was being reborn, if you would. And you mentioned, I've done five Ironman triathlons in Kona, which is a real pinnacle of success, but I do that. And I started with the run around that high school track, and each day, each week I increased the stress – not to the breaking point – but I got stronger, and stronger, and stronger, and I realized I need physical activity for my brain to function at the level I want to function at. It's a requirement.

But at the same time, my diet improved. I started working with GNC and on my supplements – the supplements we discussed entered into it. So my diet, the physical activity... and I got rid of the toxins that were involved, in terms of too much alcohol, too much anything. And then the prayer for the stress.

So my square eventually was coming back into a square, and after a year I was able to return to the most satisfying, gratifying part of my professional career. That was 20, 25 years ago, and I've been more productive, more content, more satisfied with what I'm doing than any time in my life. And now I'm in my 70s, and I must say, I came in second in my age group in the Columbus triathlon Iron Man three weeks ago.

PEGGY: Yay! Good for you!

DR MAROON: I'm allowed to brag a little bit about that.

PEGGY: Please!

DR MAROON: But it's no secret. Chuck Knoll, who was the head football coach of the Pittsburgh Steelers during the years they won all the Super Bowls, said, "Football is not complicated." He said, "It's about blocking and tackling."

Life and stress control are really not complicated. It's about the four things that we mentioned. It's about exercise, controlling the work environment, and having insight into it, avoiding environmental toxins, and controlling stress, and spirituality. If you do those four things, your life can get back into balance. It's one step at a time. It takes time, but it's possible.

PEGGY: Well, just your telling your story, which is pretty darn riveting, to go from somebody who got out of breath climbing one flight of stairs, to somebody who routinely just goes and enters the hardest triathlons... It's kind of a little lesson to all of us about the potential we may have within ourselves that we're not unleashing yet. If we put our minds to it, if we believe in ourselves enough to push ourselves a little bit more...

DR MAROON: Peggy, that's so true, and the question I ask, as a neuroscientist myself, is, "Well, what is happening? How, is behavior affected, why do we behave as we do? How do we get over things? What happens in the brain when we do these things?"

And there's a huge new field of neuroplasticity. Neuroplasticity is the brain's ability to form new connections and new fiber tracks. It used to be thought we were born with "X" number of brain cells, and we lost so many each day, and each year, until we shriveled up and died.

We now know that it's a constant regenerative process in the brain, and it's a constant modulation of new synapses and fiber tracks. So we're actually doing a study now, looking at this in patients who have burnout, and putting them into a program that involves the four factors I mentioned, plus neurofeedback using very sophisticated electroencephalography, quantitative EEG.

We're going to measure their brain fiber tracks with very sophisticated imaging before and after these interventions, to see if we can actually, for the first time, document reconnection, regeneration of these fiber tracks.

You know, I've done a lot of things. I've been very fortunate in neurosurgery, but I'm more excited about this, and what we're talking about, the process of regenerating nerve cells, and reconnecting, and neuroplasticity – of re-growing our brain, so to speak.

PEGGY: We're talking about the potential for unlimited creativity for any person, at any age, under any circumstances, if we do the right thing. And you're giving us the knowledge of what the right thing is.

I just want to review. We're going to have four sides of the square. Our first side is we must rebuild our physical health, and we know we're going to exercise to promote brain health in a powerful way. We're going to eat in a healthy way. We're going to avoid the bad, processed, sugary foods, and eat lots of healthy fats, and good veggies, and protein. We know we're going to eat better. We're not going to smoke. We're not going to over-drink... All that stuff.

Okay. The next part of our square – you know, we haven't talked enough about the second part of the square. You've mentioned that your family relationships had been neglected – you were so work-focused. Let's talk about that side of the square, human relationships.

DR MAROON: Yes, absolutely. I've given a whole lot of thought to that aspect of it. There's a superb book by a psychologist, Mihaly Csikszentmihalyi, entitled *Flow: The Ultimate Psychological Experience.* He said, "The greatest moments of our lives occur when our mind or our body is stretched to its limits in the pursuit of something both difficult and worthwhile."

I'm so blessed every day in my work. With neurosurgery, I'm pushed to my limits frequently, and the reward, the flow experience that comes from doing that successfully is huge. Doing a triathlon is the same flow experience. You're exhausted at the end, but yes, I accomplished what I wanted.

And I've thought – I've given much thought to – and we discussed this – the three most important things in life. Why am I doing this? Why am I pushing myself? And it's for that flow experience, number one, but if you think, what's really the three most important things in life? I'm going to ask your audience.

Think about it: what are the three most important things in your life? Number one, it's a healthy mind, and a healthy body. We cannot do too much for that. Without that, you know and I know that the rest of life is, like Shakespeare said, "in shallows, and in misery." So a healthy mind and a healthy body.

Number two is relationships – relationships with God, with family and friends. And I remember you shared with me your recent album. I think it's entitled, "Family and Friends," or "Friends and Family."

PEGGY: Thank you for the plug, yes. This actually – I never talk personally, but I will. This is my album, "Friends and Family" – all songs I wrote. And again, I don't usually talk personally. but this is such a personal talk. My husband had a stroke, and I am in charge of his caregiving responsibilities. And that stress was so overwhelming that I myself experienced burnout.

And one way I that I've come back is through music. When I write, I know exactly what you mean about flow, because when I write songs, I'm experiencing flow. And personally for me... It's called "Friends and Family." The title song is a tribute to my friends and family, who get me through this terrible situation I'm in. And how could I get through it without these healthy relationships? I couldn't.

DR MAROON: Well, I totally subscribe to that, and in my thinking, every day, God, family and friends is a critical portion, and I'm very blessed to be able to share my experiences with patients in a spiritual way. But let me finish the third part.

PEGGY: Yes, do.

DR MAROON: The third part is very simple: It's *carpe diem*. It's "seize the day." To be able to sit here and talk to you like we are about things that are intimate to both of us, I'm blessed to be able to do this. And I'm seizing this moment to help others, hopefully, who might learn a little bit from our own personal stories.

When it gets back to the prayer aspect of it, and stress, I operate two to three days a week, and on complicated problems with patients who are oftentimes in a lot of pain, from herniations of discs in their neck or their back, or problems in the brain.

There's no more stressful time for a person than waiting to go into the operating room, wondering what's going to happen, and what's the outcome going to be? So their cortisol level is sky-high, and we know that that reduces wound healing, prolongs hospital stay and increases complications. That's the consequence of stress and anxiety at that point.

And I found – and I'm not converting anyone, or proselytizing any specific religion – but I took care – and I describe this in the book – I took care of a priest who was the head of the Greek church in his country, and he started missionaries throughout the country, and also, was the head Abbott in Mount Athos, which is a peninsula that juts out into the Aegean Sea in northern Greece, and has been a home for monks for centuries.

And he gave me this: I'll inquire of my patients, "First of all, do you believe in God?" And I usually wear this in the operating room under my shirt.

PEGGY: Oh.

DR MAROON: And if they evince any interest at all, I'll take their hand, and I'll say a prayer. I'll say, "Can I say a prayer with you?" And I say, "Today's the day the Lord hath made. Let us rejoice and be glad in it. And with Your help, let's get Peggy back to her health, her family, and her life."

And I can only tell you I can see the cortisol level, the epinephrine and adrenalin level, the calmness come to these patients who say a 30-second prayer before going into the operating room. And probably, the most common comment I get after surgery is, "You know, Doctor, I just want to thank you for saying that prayer."

PEGGY: That's so powerful, just hearing you say that.

DR MAROON: Yeah.

PEGGY: The surgeon did not say that as he wheeled my husband into brain surgery.

DR MAROON: We have the ability in our daily work to share, in some way, spirituality, prayer, something bigger than us. I mean – je ne sais pas – I don't know what it's all about, and I struggle to some extent. But I know there's something bigger than I am, and with my Catholic upbringing – I was blessed to have a good foundation, and it's helped me through very many, many problems.

PEGGY: Well, as your talk gives us a deeper understanding of brain chemistry, we know, well, "I really don't feel like exercising. Why do I have to do exercise? Oh, I'm going to make BDNF in my brain. I'd better exercise."

We may not be used to prayer. It may feel awkward, because we're living in a time where it isn't as common to pray, or to be a member of the faith community, as it was in our grandparents' time. So it may not come naturally to us, and we may be under a time of extreme stress, and it may feel awkward, or embarrassing.

But we could say to ourselves, "You know, if I pray, Dr. Maroon says my cortisol level is going to subside. So why don't I see if I can make my cortisol level subside by prayer?" It's another way to come at it.

DR MAROON: It's another way, and it also emphasizes the importance of meditation. Prayer is a form of meditation.

PEGGY: Yes.

DR MAROON: And people who meditate, we've put them into PET scanners, and we see what areas of the brain light up, and what happens. There's a calmness that occurs with meditation, with prayer, and if you look at the areas of the world that have the most centenarians, the people who live over 100 the longest...

PEGGY: Right.

DR MAROON: ...what are some of these places? Okinawa, Sardinia, the island of Icarus in the Aegean Sea, Nicoya in Costa Rica, and the Seventh-Day Adventist community in Loma Linda, California. They have more people living over 100 than any other places in the world. Why is that?

The reason for that is they're using the epigenetic factors in the square we're talking about. They have a very healthy fish, olive oil diet, very low carbs and good, healthy fats. They work hard. They're exercising. Their environment is very pure, relatively, in terms of air and water, and they have very strong family units.

So what's the significance of the family unit, and prayer, and belief when it comes to living over a hundred? It reduces stress.

PEGGY: It reduces stress. That's our whole topic today.

DR MAROON: So that's the...

PEGGY: That's the topic.

DR MAROON: That's the thing. So again, is it complicated? It's not brain surgery.

PEGGY: You're allowed to say that.

I just want to go back to one aspect of relationships, because I had the privilege of seeing the presentation you're about to make to Harvard Medical School, and you talk marriage. Marriage, for many people, is the anchor relationship of their life, and you talk about studies of what builds up a marriage? What breaks down a marriage? What are the characteristics of how people interact with each other? Help us understand that.

DR MAROON: Yes. There's a psychologist, John Gottman, at the University of Washington, who took couples and put them in a controlled environment in which they filmed the couples.

They introduced various subjects, stressors, into the situation to see how the couple reacted to different stressors, and how they interacted. And he could predict, up to 90% of the time, which couples would subsequently end up divorced. And he enumerated several factors that are red – yellow lights that lead to red lights in a relationship.

The first is criticism. If you find in a relationship that you're constantly criticizing or being criticized, you're in for big-time trouble. Counterattack is another one, where you say something to me that I don't like, and I come right back at you and counterattack.

These kinds of interactions lead to stress. The stress leads to anxiety. The anxiety – anxiety is a protective thing. We want to get out of anxiety. What do we do to relieve ourselves of anxiety? We drink. We may get into an inappropriate relationship. We don't come home. We do a whole lot of things to get rid of the anxiety in an unhealthy way.

I think we have to be, again, mindful, as the Zen Buddhists say. You have to be mindful, you have to be aware, and you have to be in the moment. And this is very hard. It's easy to say, but it's hard to do, unless your brain is telling you what you have to do. Be aware of it.

There was a great book written in 1903 by a British writer and philosopher, James Allen. The title of the book was *As a Man Thinketh*. And it's from Proverbs 23, verse 7: "As a man thinketh, so he or she shall be."

So our thought processes control every situation in our lives, be it good or bad, in terms of the thoughts we have. You can't plant potatoes and get tomatoes.

PEGGY: No.

DR MAROON: If you have bad thoughts...

PEGGY: Right.

DR MAROON: ...bad thoughts, inappropriate thoughts, you're in an environment that's unhealthy in terms of your thinking. If you're with a peer group that's doing things that you know shouldn't be done, you're going to have problems. If you make the right choices, the moral choices, the good choices, it's going to have just the opposite effect, and you're going to blossom, and enjoy life to the fullest you can.

The important thing is that those choices not only are under our control... I mean, we make the choice. But genetically, we actually are turning our genes off for good or bad by how we think. We actually are affecting the neuroplasticity of our brain, the connections in our brain, with our thoughts.

You know, we glibly talk about the mind-body connection. Well, there's a huge connection between the mind and the body, and what happens. We know heart attacks and all the other bad things that happen. But we also know a healthy mind in a healthy body is the most important thing in life.

PEGGY: You know, you're giving us new ways to think about things that we do – as we mentioned, the exercise, we're going to think is good for our brain. Prayer, we're going to think is good for our brain. Our relationship – when maybe our husband got us a little irritated or annoyed, instead of thinking, "I just want to tell him what I think about, 'Why didn't you make the bed today?'" Whatever it was. Think, "You know what? I'm going to avoid this, because if I get into a fight, it's going to flood my brain with cortisol, and I don't need that stress right now. I don't need more – my brain has enough cortisol."

DR MAROON: That's right. You put it into much better words than I do. I get a little too technical at times. But you're right. You're exactly right.

PEGGY: It's just another way to understand – to help ourselves control ourselves, and to make healthier choices.

So we're almost done with our square. We've rebuilt our body. We've taken care of our physical health. We've improved and strengthened our relationships. We've started a spiritual relationship with our Creator to relieve stress, and to make us feel more capable of taking on challenges.

And another one that we haven't talked about, funnily enough, is work, which is the only one that was on your original diagram. What should our relationship with work be?

DR MAROON: Well, again, various studies show that 50% of the workforce in this country is fighting with a stressful work environment – commitments, schedules, demands, and it's being aware of that that's number one. Then sometimes we're caught in a bind. You know, we have to feed our family. We have to do what's necessary for our kids. So we don't have any other channels.

But again, in the work environment, if you can, be vocal in an appropriate fashion about the kinds of things that are disturbing. In the medical profession, it's just horrible at the present time, what physicians have to deal with, in terms of the electronic medical record.

PEGGY: Yeah.

DR MAROON: We spend more time putting data into a computer, not looking to the patient.

PEGGY: You got in there to help people, and you're dealing with...

DR MAROON: And it's paperwork so the insurance companies can bill appropriately.

PEGGY: Right, right. The codes and all that stuff, yeah.

DR MAROON: And many other reasons. And then, with many health systems, physicians are on a time clock. You have to see so many patients per hour. If you're not filling your quota, there are penalties.

So it's hard to escape from these kinds of daily stresses in the work environment. That's why 50% of doctors have some symptom of burnout, and feeling overwhelmed, overworked, under-producing. But being aware of it is number one. And then using the other adjuncts to modulate the stress is something that helps. There's no perfect work environment.

PEGGY: No.

DR MAROON: None. We all do things we don't want to do, but we know we have to do. But if we're aware of what we're doing, why we're doing it, and we have other outlets – like music. I love it. I mean, music tunes your brain. Literally, it tunes your brain.

PEGGY: Yeah.

DR MAROON: And it is a diversion. It brings your focus to something else that's important in your life, and takes your mind off your sore tooth. If you have a toothache and I have a toothache, we both have the same pain. But what we want to do is not focus on the pain of our toothache, if we can, but take something, an anodyne, something to relieve the pain – music for you, a bike ride or a swim for me. You know, everybody can find that in their life.

PEGGY: Okay, so I think we have our four sides of the square. I would like to keep talking with you all day, but we're reaching the end of our time, which is a shame, because I'd love to talk to you all day about this. But I don't want to end without asking you about concussions and head injuries, and so forth, because you have worked for many years with professional athletes. So what are the most important things for us to know?

DR MAROON: Well, I think, again, I have a perspective from the 1980s, when I started working with concussion problems, to the present time, and I've seen a huge evolution in care and recognition of the problem.

Initially, when we began, you know, it was, "How many fingers do you see?", and a little ammonia chloride, smelling salts under the nose, and they went back into the game. Now there's nothing farther from the truth than that, and we realize that the major problem with concussions is returning before the brain has had time to heal.

Let me explain. If you get a splinter under your finger, what happens to your finger? It gets red, hot, tender and swollen. That's the body's innate immune response to protect the body. If you get hit in the head, what happens to the brain? The cells in the brain called microglia, that you're familiar with, release the same chemicals that cause the red, hot, tender and swollen reaction in your finger.

After a period of time – a week, two weeks or so – those chemicals dissipate, and BDNF kicks in to reduce the inflammation, and to heal the brain and repair the cells.

If you get hit in that interval before the brain gets into the healing process, then it's like a brush fire in a dry forest. You can get cascading deterioration of function, including headaches, and nausea, and visual and vestibular problems, balance problems.

So probably the most important thing is, number one, a single concussion by itself, in the great majority of cases, is not a permanent injury. I've had seven concussions playing football at the University of Indiana. You know, one crash with a pad, bus, or a motorcycle – yes, can do terrible damage. But the concussions that we see in sports are not, in themselves, life-changing or life-altering in the vast, vast majority of cases. The important thing is they be managed properly.

We designed a test called "Impact," which is a neurocognitive test now in use. We've tested 13 million kids baseline with this test, before they participate in contact sports. If there's a concussion, or concussive episode, they're retested. They don't return to sports until they've come back to their baseline as one of the things necessary to return.

So the knowledge, the awareness has been hugely beneficial, and I think still sports are the most important thing that kids can do. The lack of it is contributing to the obesity epidemic.

General MacArthur said it best. He has a plaque at West Point, where he was the commandant, that faces the playing fields – the baseball, the soccer, the football fields – and it says, "On the fields of friendly strife are sown the seeds that, on other days and on other fields, will lead to victory."

"On the fields of friendly strife" – the stress – Again, the stress that you learn. You don't quit. You get up when you fall. You move on. You have teamwork. There's loyalty. These are all qualities you get from sports, and in particular, football. I wouldn't be sitting here today with you if I did not play youth football, because it completely changed my life in the environment that I was raised in.

So my take on it is, I encourage controlled sports by coaches who understand the problem, and parents who get involved themselves. But I don't think there's anything better that a young boy or a young girl can do. We talk about concussions in football. Girls' soccer has a higher, or at least as high, a rate of incidents of concussions as male football. But it's very little talked about, soccer.

PEGGY: That's true.

DR MAROON: But we need to protect the brains of all these kids, and that's what we're all about.

PEGGY: What you're saying is you sometimes see permanent injury if people return to play too soon; that, just as in exercise there's a natural healing process that happens to our brain through exercise. There's a natural process that happens when our brain is injured, that we heal through rest. Is that correct?

DR MAROON: To rest, and now we used to put people at complete bed rest – complete rest – cocoon them, so to speak, after a concussion.

PEGGY: Right.

DR MAROON: We now know that's not the right approach. We encourage exercise, as long as it doesn't reproduce the symptoms for the same reason we've talked about, in terms of regenerating the growth factors in the brain.

PEGGY: The healthy stress, but not over into the cortisol-producing stress.

DR MAROON: Exactly, exactly.

PEGGY: Okay, so I think that gives us a good, basic understanding of current knowledge of dealing with concussions, so thank you for that.

Thank you for everything. We've learned so much. It's such a rich conversation. There's so much to absorb here. Thank you.

DR MAROON: Well, it's my pleasure. I enjoy sharing this, because, I mean, I get letters like you do. This has made a big difference to me, and Sanjay Gupta, one of the endorsers of the book, basically said the same thing. He said he's gotten something from this, as knowledgeable as he is. So I love sharing it, and I appreciate the opportunity, Peggy.

PEGGY: Thank you so much for watching, and I hope you get a chance to read Dr. Maroon's book, *Square One*, and learn more about his wisdom, and the four sides of the square to keep your life in balance, and keep your brain healthy. So thank you, and good luck.

Interview with Norman Doidge, M.D.

PEGGY SARLIN: Hello, I'm Peggy Sarlin, and today I'm in Toronto, Canada with Dr. Norman Doidge, the best-selling author of *The Brain's Way of Healing* and *The Brain That Changes Itself.*

These books have helped millions of people understand the concept of neuroplasticity, the ability of the brain to grow new cells and create new networks. And that turns out to be enormously important for healing a very broad spectrum of problems, ranging from learning disorders, to traumatic brain injury, to Parkinson's, and potentially to Alzheimer's and dementia.

Dr. Doidge is a psychiatrist and a psychoanalyst with the University of Toronto and Columbia University in New York. He has traveled the world to find new techniques to stimulate neuroplasticity in your brain. And this is really staggering stuff. It can create miracles, as you're going to hear. So welcome, Dr. Doidge.

DR DOIDGE: It's great to be here.

PEGGY: So Doctor, your books describe techniques that manipulate energy in the body to create neuroplasticity in the brain. Why don't we start out by understanding what neuroplasticity is?

DR DOIDGE: Sure. It's a property of the brain that allows it to change its structure, its physical structure, and its function in response to mental experience and activity.

So what you do, what you experience, what you think, even what you imagine can actually change your brain structure. And what we've been doing in the last while is using our understanding of plasticity to help people with various kinds of brain problems.

PEGGY: When you say it changes the structure, if we're going to look at imagery of a brain, it's going to look different after you've done these techniques that we're going to describe today. The brain is actually physically going to change.

DR DOIDGE: Yes, yeah.

PEGGY: Okay, that's exciting stuff.

DR DOIDGE: At many different levels. In small parts of the brain, one can actually grow new cells, and it turns out that those small parts of the brain are actually relevant for Alzheimer's. Throughout the brain, through the rest of the brain, you can change the connectivity between the cells. You can grow new connections, or prune away various other connections to actually change the networks in the brain.

PEGGY: Well, you talked about small areas of the brain, so I'm assuming you're talking about the hippocampus, among others.

DR DOIDGE: Yes.

PEGGY: I mention it because I think a lot of people who are watching know that the hippocampus is the place where Alzheimer's tends to begin. So we can use neuroplastic techniques to encourage new health, new cells in the hippocampus.

DR DOIDGE: Yes, and I want to emphasize that neuroplasticity isn't something we just use in the course of illness. Neuroplasticity is the modus operandi of the brain, and the reason that we're discovering it now is in part because we now have the technology to actually do microscopic movies, and we can see the brain changing.

But the brain's always been plastic, and everything you do in one way or another changes the structure of your brain. But we didn't appreciate that, because the model people had of the brain for the last 400 years was that the brain was like a machine.

Over and over, what human beings have done to come to terms with the complexity of the brain is to try to have some kind of metaphor for the brain. Machines were very impressive to people 400 years ago, and so they started to talk about the brain as a hydraulic machine.

And then, when electricity developed, they started to talk about the brain as though it was an electrical machine. And we still speak of things like circuits in the brain.

And now people are increasingly talking about it as though it's a computer. But that's wrong. The brain is not an inanimate machine. Machines do many glorious things, but they don't grow new parts or new connectivities when they're damaged.

So the machine metaphor has actually gotten in the way of our understanding of the brain. We have to understand the brain on its own terms.

PEGGY: So understand the brain in its own terms... This basic concept of neuroplasticity, when we're dealing with a disorder, a brain disorder or a brain problem, kind of works on the premise that if, let's say, the bridge is washed out on one part of the brain, then you can reroute and go elsewhere, and get function back. Is that a proper way to say it?

DR DOIDGE: Often, you can. Maybe not always, because, you know, no two strokes are identical.

PEGGY: Yes.

DR DOIDGE: No two traumatic brain injuries are identical. And you need the ability to pay attention to make new circuits. But if you have that, you often can basically perform activities, and get other brain areas to take over from the areas that have been damaged.

For instance, there's a fantastic treatment for stroke called constraint-induced therapy. As an example, when a person has had a stroke and can't use their right hand, what they will tend to do is increasingly use their left hand. It's a use-it-or-lose-it brain, and that may strengthen the circuitry that is governing the left hand. But in the meantime, the right hand, which is already damaged, will completely wither, because it's a use-it-or-lose-it brain.

So what the therapist will do in that treatment is to actually take the hand you want to use, put it in a cast so you can't use it, and then incrementally retrain the affected arm.

And when they do brain scans on these people, what they find is that areas in the brain adjacent to where there is the lesion or cell death from the stroke will take over, or sometimes, areas in the opposite hemisphere, mirror areas in the opposite hemisphere will start to process the activity so that this hand can move.

It doesn't move quite as well as it originally did, but there are 500 studies now showing that this treatment is a powerful intervention, and that's a great example of neuroplasticity in action.

PEGGY: That's not a machine. If your dishwasher broke down, I could not reconstitute, could not totally change the way it works.

DR DOIDGE: Not a lot of dishwashers.

PEGGY: But the brain works the way you just described it.

Many of these techniques that you write about involve manipulating energy in the body. And I think most of us who aren't doctors don't walk around thinking of our bodies as electrical systems, as energy units. So can we start by understanding a little bit about that – how our brains are internally making energy?

DR DOIDGE: Sure. The brain does work, and that requires energy. And the brain actually uses about 20% of your energy consumption, even though it's only several percentage points – two or three percent – of your body weight, perhaps. So it really punches above its weight in the consumption of energy.

For the last number of years, there's been a tremendous emphasis on brain chemistry. People think of brain problems, and they think of advertisements they've heard that tell them that depression is a chemical disease, or Parkinson's is a chemical disease. And we focus very, very much on brain chemistry. And of course, there is brain chemistry, and it is important.

But the way brain cells connect globally with each other is by electrical signals or spikes. Brain chemistry works in between neurons. It works very locally and microscopically. But your brain works by transmitting signals, from neuron to neuron, and into the body, and into your muscles so that they contract, and so on.

Now, one of the very neat things about the brain is that it has these windows to the outside world, which are our sense organs. And our sense organs actually will take energy from the outside world, and convert it into something electrical.

So your eyes will take photons, and they convert it into electrical signals. Your ears will take soundwaves, and convert them into electrical signals in the brain.

These sense organs are what are called transducers in engineering, or even in biology. They take energy of one form and convert it into energy of another form. They also take patterns of energy of one form, and convert it to patterns of energy in another form.

For example, we're talking into microphones right now. They are transducers. They're taking soundwaves and making them into an electrical signal, which then comes out of a speaker, which is also a transducer, which will take an electrical signal, and make it into a sound wave.

Now, our sense organs are transducers, and what we can do is use the energy patterns around us to sculpt the plastic brain, if we know what we're doing.

I didn't set out to emphasize energy, but after my first book, which tried to establish that neuroplasticity is clinically important and culturally important, and that culture shapes our brains, and that we can use plasticity for all sorts of medical purposes... I started to explore neuroplasticity throughout the world, and the theme that kept coming up over and over again was that people were finding that energy is a great pathway to noninvasively influence brain structure.

I want to emphasize that. "Noninvasively" is important, because invasive medical procedures have a lot of potential risk.

We can now get inside the deepest part of the brain, for instance, through the tongue. By stimulating the tongue with certain electrical patterns, we can get into the brain stem. And the brain stem is a massive control center for the brain and the body, and we influence that.

We can get into the brain and influence it with light, and with sound, and even with movement, if we know what we're doing.

It turns out that we tended to think of the brain as though it's buried deep inside your head, and the only way to get to it is either through drugs in the bloodstream – which are a very blunt instrument, because they go through the entire body – or by cracking open a skull in surgery.

What I emphasize is getting at the brain in the natural way. Because really, it's only in anatomy textbooks that your brain is cut off or separate from the body. In physiology textbooks and in reality, your brain is seamlessly connected to your body and your sense organs, which are seamlessly connected to the energy of the outside world.

And so we can influence the brain in a very natural way, noninvasively. Sometimes very remarkably.

PEGGY: That's very exciting stuff, and that's what we're going to get into. But just to return for a minute to the fact that you said there's been a lot of emphasis on brain chemistry, but now we're looking at brain energy.

We're looking at the fact that the brain communicates through electrical signals. And is it generally a component, if there's a brain disorder, that there is an electrical problem? That there's an energy problem going on in the brain? Is that a common component of a lot of brain dysfunction?

DR DOIDGE: It's important in a number of medical conditions. One of the things I found that happens in many brain problems is that the signaling is irregular, in some ways. People have heard of irregular signals when they think of heart problems. They know that there is such a thing as arrhythmia. Sometimes the heart fires too quickly, or too slowly, or irregularly.

Well, what I found as I started to review things is that there are many brain problems where the signaling is off, if you will, or it's asynchronous. So it gives rise to what I call a noisy brain.

PEGGY: Did you make up that term?

DR DOIDGE: Yes.

PEGGY: The noisy brain. I like it.

DR DOIDGE: Okay, let me give you an example. This is just one example among many. We used to think, for instance, that if a person lost the use of their right hand in a stroke, and they lost 90% of the function of that hand, that 90% of the cells governing movement and sensation in that hand – or the tracks leading from those cells to the hand – must be damaged.

But as I started to spend a lot of time looking at the electrical firing patterns in a number of conditions, what I found was this: Some cells are dead. But often, cells adjacent to those dead cells are in some way metabolically compromised, or sick.

And sick cells don't necessarily fall silent completely. Rather, what they may do is fire at the wrong rate. And then there are healthy cells that are connected to those sick cells, and they are getting irregular signals, and they can't use those signals.

So you've got some dead cells, some sick cells which are of no use, and then healthy cells receiving junk data, and they'll send out junk data. If that's the case, what we find you can do is you can try to do something to help those sick cells, and you can also re-synchronize the firing of the brain by all sorts of ways of influencing the brain, using energy patterns, or things like neuro-feedback, which is another technique you can use to restore the normal firing.

And suddenly, someone who has had 90% loss of function might get a lot of that function back, because really, only a few of the cells are dead – not nearly as many as we feared.

The other thing to keep in mind is there are so many cells in the brain that you actually can afford to lose some, if they're in certain places. We're all losing some.

The most important thing is that the signaling is clear, that it's not noisy, which means that the signals that your brain makes can stand out against the background activity in the brain, so that the signals are clear and sharp. So re-synchronizing the noisy brain turns out to be a great way to improve the brain in a number of conditions.

PEGGY: Would Alzheimer's be one of them, do you think?

DR DOIDGE: It might be helpful. You know, what I found as I started to explore so many different neuroplastic interventions was... well, here's how it came to me in practice: I wrote a book on the brain, and how it could heal more than we thought, and then many people who had had traumatic brain injuries naturally contacted me. And I got more and more interested in that subject, to see if injured brains could be helped.

And the overwhelming majority of people with traumatic brain injury are told they have a concussion or an injury. They go to the doctor, and they're told, "You've got an 80% chance of recovering." And some people do recover.

But what about the 20% who don't recover? Well, they're told to rest and wait it out. In fact, we really don't have very much in mainstream medicine for them except pray, if they don't get better.

I was starting to hear about all these different interventions. And suddenly, there was an embarrassment of riches of different things that you could try for traumatic brain injury. I tried to develop it – just order it in my head, because people who've had traumatic brain injuries are typically unemployed. They're disabled. I mean, they don't have a lot of money.

So I tried to figure out, well, what intervention would be best for this particular person, or that? And I realized that different interventions worked at different levels. So I developed these five stages of neuroplastic healing.

Number one – the first phase – is to address general cellular health. In many brain problems, and Alzheimer's is definitely one of them, there are things that are going wrong in the cells. So that's always the first thing I would address.

And even in traumatic brain injury, a few days after the injury there's a lot of toxicity in the brain that's actually killing cells. Sometimes a person can be okay for a window of time, and then they actually get worse. So cellular health is always very important to address. And it's especially important in Alzheimer's that we get back to that.

The next step – and the kinds of interventions, by the way, that deal with cellular health – include light. Light is one of them. Hyperbaric oxygen is another one; making sure that the person doesn't have any mineral deficits, various kinds of deficits; getting rid of toxicities; dietary interventions. Dietary interventions actually are huge, because so many people are sensitive to so many things.

Addressing the gut as a way to get to the brain is another one, because if you have a leaky gut, then substances can trigger the immune system and get into the brain. So that's the first priority: cellular health.

The next stage is what I call "neural stimulation." We've said it's a use-it-or-lose-it brain, and one of the things that happens in the brain is that, whenever there's any injury, one of the defenses is for that circuitry and the related circuitry to actually go dormant.

That's a very common protective mechanism in biology. If something's not working, you don't want to be using up all of your energy to do it. Imagine a circuit's noisy and not functioning properly. So dormancy is a huge thing that happens.

For instance, when a person has a stroke, after the initial bleed or clot, the body has to reabsorb the blood, and there's a lot of chemical chaos in the brain after every stroke.

PEGGY: Yes.

DR DOIDGE: And even if the stroke's in a small area, the chemical chaos kind of spreads through the brain, and the brain doesn't function all that well. If you try to move your hand, it won't work properly. You keep trying, and if it doesn't work, the brain learns that it's not working.

PEGGY: It's pointless.

DR DOIDGE: And the circuitry actually kind of goes dormant. That's called "learned non-use." People who have learned non-use just think that it must be brain damage. But actually, some of it is learned.

It's valuable knowing that there is learned non-use, not only in stroke, but to some degree in Parkinson's, and you can get some of it in MS – and what the clinicians have got to do is find ways to stimulate that circuitry. Some of it can be exercise, there are many different ways we do it. Some of it can be with sound. Some of it can be with neuro-feedback, which, again, requires a whole explanation. But neuro-stimulation is the next thing I tend to address.

Then I've already mentioned the noisy brain. It figures in so many conditions, not just epilepsy. Parts of Parkinson's, sometimes stroke, learning disorders, autism, aspects of Alzheimer's, probably... these conditions show brains that aren't firing synchronously properly. So the next thing to do is to resynchronize the firing.

The next phase is something I call "neuro-relaxation," and it doesn't occur all the time. But one of the things I noticed with certain treatments – for instance, the sound treatment, sometimes the light treatments, sometimes the electrical stimulation on the tongue to resynchronize the brain stem – is that patients would suddenly start sleeping for 16, 18 hours a day for a number of days.

I label that as a phase, because that's when the brain is doing lots and lots of recovery. And you don't want to interrupt that sleep. You don't want to treat that sleep as though it's pathological.

The final stage is neuro-differentiation, and that is a stage where the brain learns to make new distinctions. As I said, it's a use-it-or-lose-it brain. Imagine you had a stroke... or here's another example: Let's say a child was born spastic, with cerebral palsy, and they couldn't move their limbs.

PEGGY: Okay.

DR DOIDGE: Well it happens that one of the ways we actually form our brain maps is by movement. We know that babies often don't distinguish each of their fingers. And gradually they learn, by moving them at different times, to distinguish them. And as they move their fingers at different times, that's how the brain maps differentiate.

We know this from all sorts of brain scans: If you were to tape your fingers together and move them all together at the same time, you would not have a brain map for each individual finger.

PEGGY: Okay.

DR DOIDGE: You would just have a map for this mitt. So kids with cerebral palsy don't even develop their brain maps properly, which means if we could start moving their fingers, help them eliminate the spasticity – which sometimes, we can – and move them differently, we can actually build up brain maps.

Now after a stroke or any brain problem where you are not using a function, the use-it-or-lose-it brain maps start to de-differentiate. The distinctions, let's say, between the fingers, if that would be the example, start to blur and you end up with a kind of club hand.

PEGGY: Right.

DR DOIDGE: So one of the final things we do for any brain that's been injured is we re-differentiate things. And that can go for movements, speech, various forms of learning to differentiate body states.

Neuro-differentiations are really powerful. Even brain exercises, to some degree, can help with neuro-differentiation. But some of the various body work that people do develops neuro-differentiation.

PEGGY: Okay, so let's start going into some of the techniques that people might find they can use on their family member. Light. You mentioned light. How is light going to rewire our brain?

DR DOIDGE: In the early 60s, some discoveries were made about laser lights. Now, laser lights, when we hear that term, we often think of the power of light to destroy. You think of the James Bond movie...

PEGGY: Right.

DR DOIDGE: ...and Goldfinger about to split Mr. Bond in half.

PEGGY: Right.

DR DOIDGE: Those are hot lasers. They burn flesh. But there are other kinds of laser lights which are sometimes called "cold lasers." They're not really cold. They're just not hot. And it was discovered by scientists that they actually can help healing. Originally, they did experiments, and they showed that animals that had wounds could be healed with these kinds of lasers, or, in some of them, hair could grow.

So people increasingly started to use these lights for biomechanical problems. Although all the lasers were invented in North America, a lot of this was studied in Eastern Europe where they had less of an emphasis, perhaps, on chemicals and drugs.

They started shining light on things like E. coli – small organisms – and they found that light could do many, many things. They found that light could actually help the production of DNA. It could lower inflammation in bodies. It could eliminate pain.

So people started using light for the body. There's one case I described where one of the physicians was using it for someone who had suffered a neck injury in a car accident. The physician put light on the back of his neck. That man also had had a stroke which narrowed his field of vision.

And in the course of his treatment for his sore neck, his field of vision, which was like a keyhole, started to expand. And the physician realized, "My goodness, I'm also very, very close to the occipital cortex, the part of the brain that processes vision. Maybe light is actually helping vision."

And a number of clinicians started increasingly using light for things like migraine headaches, and ultimately for traumatic brain injuries.

What we believe is happening here is that there are certain specific frequencies that are in these lasers that promote healing and decrease inflammation. And they also influence the mitochondria, which are the powerhouses in the cell, so to speak. They produce the energy to re-energize.

So the cell is extremely dependent on the mitochondria. It's like the power source in the cell that enables it to do its other work. Cells are always in the state of repair, and many of them are in a growth state.

We now know, in fact, that light can be used to help a number of people with traumatic brain injury, for instance. And it's been used in some cases to help stroke as well, I think by helping the cells to get to the point where they can function again properly.

So light is a general cellular intervention, but it also leads to neuro-stimulation of those circuits.

PEGGY: Let's clarify. When we're talking about light here, we're talking specifically about this cold laser.

DR DOIDGE: Cold laser, but LED lights at the right frequency will also do it. Compared to the typical LED lights, the lasers can go deeper into the body, maybe 7, 10 cm deeper. You can also get the same effect with LED lights that are well-tuned to these healing frequencies, but they don't go as deep into the body.

PEGGY: We can shine a cold laser into the brain, and cool down inflammation, right? Because inflammation is characteristic...

DR DOIDGE: We can cool down pathological inflammation. That's the beauty of it. If your body is doing normal inflammation, that's a wonderful, welcome thing. But in many brain problems – something like MS, aspects of Alzheimer's, perhaps, but whenever there's been a bleed, or a stroke – there often is a chronic inflammatory process, which ends up being destructive.

It's almost like inflammation starts, and it doesn't go through to completion, and it becomes chronic. And beautifully – or luckily, anyway – that's the process that low-intensity lasers and lights can push through to the end.

PEGGY: I should mention that Dr. Dale Bredesen, whom I recently interviewed, has divided Alzheimer's into three types. The first type is inflammatory, the inflamed brain is characteristic of Alzheimer's. So having this non-pharmaceutical way to get deep into the brain, and potentially cool down inflammation, seems extremely promising. That's what it seems like.

DR DOIDGE: I would put it in the promising category.

PEGGY: Yes, in the promising category.

DR DOIDGE: There are some studies that are ongoing now. They're just starting up in Toronto. There were animal studies that were done in Australia that showed improvements. And if you're looking at rats and mice, you know, you don't have very deep to go to get into the brain.

There were welcome changes pathologically in the brains of those animals, and they performed better after the light therapy. We have to see if that will also work on human beings.

But I do want to say, because the brain is complicated, that I don't believe in the following statement – the following question: What is the appropriate treatment for Brain Condition X? As though there's one treatment that matches a disorder. Let me explain why that is.

In medicine there is low-hanging fruit and high-hanging fruit, and we've gotten a lot of the low-hanging fruit.

PEGGY: Right.

DR DOIDGE: And low-hanging fruit are things similar to a snake bite, where there's one antidote for it, and if you give the person that, they get better. It's as though it's a kind of linear system.

PEGGY: Right.

DR DOIDGE: We know where there's a breakdown, and what the problem is. In many of the conditions in medicine that are yet to be solved, we're dealing with very, very complex problems, with many multiple, reciprocal interactions, and each of them is different.

Dr. Bredesen's shown that there are multiple paths to Alzheimer's, for instance. So it stands to reason that there would be different approaches to each of them. And what we know from his work, and what I find in my work, is that most people with a brain problem need multiple approaches. That's where the phases of neuro-plastic healing may be helpful, because it tells us, are we addressing these various things?

In Alzheimer's, we know there are many biochemical things going wrong. There are hormonal things. There are inflammatory problems, etc. And the light may play a role as being part of the protocol.

PEGGY: If somebody is watching this and they say, "Oh, that sounds like it might be promising" – where do they go? Where do they find somebody to treat their brain with cold lasers?

DR DOIDGE: Well, a lot of what's happening in Toronto, in Boston, in Israel, is at a research level. Lights in general are very, very safe. There are a few mistakes people can make with lights, there are some places where you shouldn't put them, and so on.

And you don't necessarily need lasers. You can do LEDs; make them very safe. I would always work with your physician, someone who knows you. In Toronto, Meditech is one place that has done a lot of work with light – not so much for dementia, but they've done a lot of work with traumatic brain injury.

Anita Saltmarche is here in Toronto. She participated with Margaret Naeser in one of the very first studies. I think it was the first study, actually, of head injury and light in human beings. So these are some people to try, and also here in Toronto there's a manufacturer of something called "Vielight," and people are trying that for a lot of brain problems.

PEGGY: Can you spell that for us?

DR DOIDGE: I think it's V-I-E-L-I-G-H-T. So there are several manufacturers. There are manufacturers throughout the world. You've got to really check this out, because it's very easy to make cheap lights, sell them inexpensively, but they're not necessarily reliable.

But for traumatic brain injury, I would say they should certainly work with someone who's got a lot of experience with it. And to begin with, make sure the diagnosis is correct. Work with your own physician. And then in some cases, you might buy a home light, after you've already seen an expert, and work with that.

PEGGY: Just to talk a little bit about light as medicine, you describe the incident in your book in which Florence Nightingale discovered that when she brought soldiers out into the courtyard and they got sunshine, they got better than the soldiers who were patients inside the hospital.

Is this something we should keep in mind in general, in terms of staying healthy, or dealing with somebody who might be sick in some ways – the capacity of sunlight to heal?

DR DOIDGE: Well, I think so. I think so. The great problem with modern life is that science and technology have put us in all sorts of artificial conditions. There's millions of years of evolution of animals that accustom them to being in a particular environment, and that environment included a lot of time spent in sunlight. And it's not just because sunlight is helpful with things like Vitamin D. There are many reasons why sunlight is helpful. We spend our time with artificial light.

You know, the Florence Nightingale story is great, because, as I recall, she was a nurse in the Crimean War, and it was just an observation she made – that the patients who had wounds on the battlefield did better than people who were in various kinds of tents. And she had a tremendous impact on the design of hospitals in England and other places.

In the old days, they would design a hospital so everyone had access to natural light. With the discovery of the light bulb, and Edison's work, and so on, people assumed that the light bulb invention would have all of the key frequencies or components that natural light did. So they eliminated windows in hospitals, or...

PEGGY: And courtyards.

DR DOIDGE: ...and all of that sort of stuff. And that was a huge mistake, because the artificial light, the typical artificial light doesn't have in it what natural light does.

The other thing that happened was that light was very frequently used as a treatment for things like tuberculosis and things like smallpox, as I recall. And there was a tremendous amount of pollution in places like Boston and London from coal production. And kids couldn't get better, so they would sometimes put them on boats and take them out so that they would get light to heal them.

People also used to go to various places in the Alps for exposure to light for things like tuberculosis. It didn't always work, but it did work sometimes.

With the development of antibiotics, people forgot about light as a therapy. And with people working very long hours inside, they forget about it in their everyday life.

So look: You're in the doldrums. You're living in New York City. It's February and I say, "Okay, I'm giving you a holiday in the Bahamas." And you feel good. Your cells start singing, because they're telling you something: that you need that light.

PEGGY: We need light. I think that's a good thing in general to keep in mind. We need light. Our bodies are designed to function well with sunlight.

But we've done light. Let's talk about sound. How do you use sound intervention?

DR DOIDGE: Let me take an extreme example of a very challenging situation. Let's talk about something like autism, but what I'm saying also applies to many learning disorders.

Autism, again, is one of these complex disorders, so that no two kids with autism are identical, and you have to address all the stages, in my opinion, of neuroplastic healing to get a chance at improvement.

But this is something that's very well-known: The majority of kids with autism are actually hypersensitive to sound. So those very noisy walkways in airports, for instance, or escalators...

PEGGY: Right.

DR DOIDGE: ...or certain machine sounds really trouble those kids, and they're covering their ears all the time, and often screaming. There's a number of sounds that really trouble those kids. And there are so many symptoms in autism that clinicians used to think, "Well, that's just part of the autistic package in many, many kids, but it couldn't be all that important."

Well, it turns out it's actually really important, sound sensitivities. When you walk into a party and there are a lot of people there, it's kind of booming, buzzing confusion, and there's just kind of a rumble. You can't make it out. But over time, you start to focus on individual conversations. There's some people that are talking about religion here, and politics here, and romance here...

What's happening is that, just as in a camera, there's a zoom lens in your ear. There's something like an auditory zoom that can focus in on the frequencies of human speech. But in autistic kids, many of them with sound sensitivities, or in kids with sensory integration disorder, or in kids with auditory processing disorders, that auditory zoom is often not working very well.

For human beings – in fact, for all animals – there are certain frequencies with which we communicate with other human beings, and in those frequencies, most people are pretty comfortable. We evolved to be comfortable in those frequencies, the frequencies of human speech.

But there are other frequencies. Those are sounds that, for instance, predators, animals that kill us, make, and those make us very anxious, for fight or flight reasons. We don't want animals that prey on us to be able to hear our communication frequencies...

PEGGY: Right.

DR DOIDGE: ...and we are really sensitive to the sounds they make.

Now, if you think about going to the movies, and if there's a monster coming on the screen... if there's an alien on the screen... if there's a shark – the music is always very, very low. You know, it's just very, very frightening to hear that low sound. If a person is possessed by an alien, you'll forgive me, but...(making low, scratchy tones) in some very low, frightening sound.

Now, autistic kids are not hearing human speech sounds which are calming to us. They are often hearing sounds which are very threatening, and so they're covering their ears to block out the sound, but also to try to regulate their fear and their terror. That's really, really important to understand.

A French doctor named Alfred Tomatis made a series of discoveries, and one of them was that you could actually train up an auditory zoom by taking certain kinds of music and modifying it so that, at times, you're triggering something they're comfortable with, and then something they're uncomfortable with.

So this is now part of the package of treatment for autism. It's not widely known, but I have definitely seen severe cases of autistic children who go to becoming mild. And occasionally – not always, but at times – I've seen kids who are significantly autistic fall off the spectrum.

There are cases of kids who were autistic who do fall off the spectrum, and there are some who don't. Most people, most parents are told, "Autism is genetic. There's nothing you can do about it. Be mature as a parent, and adapt to it."

But there are more and more case histories of people who are very well diagnosed who make significant improvements with different kinds of interventions, and occasionally even fall off the spectrum.

What happens in these situations is that the kid will come to a place called The Listening Center. That's one of the places that does this in North America – the one that I've studied the most. And they start listening to modified music. The therapists at the center tend to work with Mozart – there's a number of reasons for that, but it's higher frequencies that kind of lay the groundwork for human speech.

And then they fiddle with it. They modify the music. And as they start to develop the auditory zoom – and sometimes it can happen in several days – kids will do amazing things. They will turn to their father for the first time and hug him. And their speech will improve, and they lose their sound sensitivities.

What's happening here is the following. It's complicated, but it's really important to know.

When you're in a fight or flight mode, you really turn off what's called "the social engagement system." The social engagement system is the system that allows us to modulate our speech, to look people in the eye, to hear the frequencies of human speech, amongst other things.

If you want to connect with people, all of those things have to be done. If you're constantly in fight or flight mode because of the sound, you will turn off the social engagement system.

This is such an important fact, because some people will say that the essence of autism is the inability to model other minds. And if that's the case, how is it possible that a kid listening to music can, within several days, suddenly express love for their parent?

What that tells us is they had that capacity. And by the way, some parents sense that. They had that capacity, but it was constantly being turned off because they were in fight or flight because of the ear problem.

And you can use this to help kids with auditory or attention problems. Some attention problems are actually listening problems and auditory processing problems. You can use it for a range of problems.

There are patients I've seen who had traumatic brain injury. By the way, they often will develop hypersensitivity to sound, and sound can be an important component of their treatment. And there are other things you can do with sound, too.

But again, what's happening here? We're using patterns of information contained in energy to modify the brain circuitry and re-sculpt it, build new processers, in some ways, silence the noisy brain so that the brain can function at capacity.

PEGGY: This is a great example of using energy to promote neuroplasticity, because you're not giving anybody a pill. It's not a pharmaceutical drug. You're having them listen to music and/or sounds in ways that are going to enable them to activate their auditory zoom. It's like they're not hearing the soundtrack of "Jaws" going in their mind all the time.

DR DOIDGE: Kind of – yeah. Or very frequently, you're right.

PEGGY: Right, so that I can't focus on you. I'm too busy being scared about this impending shark.

DR DOIDGE: And not even understanding why I'm so scared, which is also disorienting and even frightening.

PEGGY: Right, just your heart...

DR DOIDGE: And why is nobody else scared? Why am I scared? There are so many things that those children are going through. You see, there are some medications we have in medicine that actually go in there and fix a problem, like an antibiotic, when it's working and used appropriately, and not overused.

PEGGY: Right.

DR DOIDGE: But most of the medications in psychiatry and neurology don't fix the problem. They're not even designed to fix the problem. The model that people have is "the system is broken." The brain is broken. You hear that phrase. It's a machine, and it's broken.

And so what they're doing is they have a medication that props up the failing system. But stop the medication, forget your dose, and the symptoms and the problem return.

What's beautiful about the kind of intervention I've described is that you're actually training the brain. And once they get it properly differentiated, if there is an element of neuro-differentiation in their auditory cortex with this kind of training, they learn to properly modulate or neuro-modulate their emotions, because their fight/flight system isn't always being turned on inappropriately.

It's not as though they have to walk around listing to music all day long. The therapy is typically something like 15 days.

PEGGY: Really!

DR DOIDGE: And then you might wait for a number of months, and then do another session, and then maybe once a year for a few years. But basically that's it. In those cases, I don't even want to say the problem is fixed, because that's kind of a machine metaphor.

PEGGY: Right.

DR DOIDGE: Their brain grows out of the problem, or it accesses its potential, or it heals itself. And I think healing is an appropriate word here. Healing comes from an old English word, and it really means to make "whole again." I think that's what's happening there.

PEGGY: So we've got sound. We've got light. And another recommendation you discuss in the book is the possibility of online programming to activate certain brain patterns to encourage new neuroplasticity, I guess, in positive ways. Tell us, are there programs you recommend? Who is it appropriate for?

DR DOIDGE: Yeah. It really does come down to which programs are well-studied. Often one reads in the papers these headlines: "Brain Exercises..." or usually they'll say something like, "Brain Games of No Use."

These are based on studies which, I must say, are deeply problematic, because they put together apples and oranges and figs and spoiled apples and spoiled figs... They just lump them all together. Anything that has to do with the brain and some kind of computer is called a brain game or exercise.

Once plasticity was discovered, many people started throwing the word around and rebranding old-fashioned kinds of brain games as though they were effective. And they're not all equal.

I'll tell you about one that I've studied closely, the Brain HQ exercises. And I have no financial involvement with this in any way, but I happened to be there when the company was two people in a living room. And one of the people in the living room was arguably one of the leading scientists in the world, Michael Merzenich, who had done so much to persuade skeptical scientists that the brain is plastic.

He was interested in neurological and psychiatric problems. He was a prophet in San Francisco [University of California, San Francisco], and there's now over 150 studies, good studies that show that Brain HQ is helpful for age-related cognitive decline and many other brain problems.

The first thing people say whenever you talk about brain exercises is, "Okay great. So you can get good at the brain exercise. But does it generalize?"

Yes, it does generalize. It generalizes to everyday life. For instance, they've got a visual brain exercise which a number of studies have shown that if you give it to elderly people, they have fewer car accidents. They can process things happening in real time much faster. That is generalization.

And they followed many people, for instance, who were elderly in a hugely expensive study sponsored by NIH at many different hospitals, and showed that the elderly people who did the exercises were better in managing everyday life.

Brain exercises like this work by, I believe, stimulating pathways and neuro-differentiation. But this has been put together by a team of neuro-scientists. It's not the same as some person just doing an app with a game.

Similar exercises are being studied all over the world. Now in Toronto they're being studied for traumatic brain injury. Again, no two injuries are the same. So in some cases, I don't recommend brain exercises for traumatic brain injury. I would recommend addressing other things first, and then later I will suggest brain exercises.

But early on, a person might just get a headache. I believe you've got to address some of the cellular things that are happening first, and then you can get into neuro-stimulation.

PEGGY: So if we're not dealing with traumatic brain injury, but we're dealing with just age-related cognitive decline, senior moments, or maybe even the beginning of Alzheimer's, this kind of brain exercise could be beneficial.

DR DOIDGE: Well, let's differentiate those two. First, age-related cognitive decline: It's a use-it-or-lose-it brain, and as most of us hit middle-age, we go to a party and we're introduced to three people, and we swear we're going to remember their names, and we just can't hold onto it.

And increasingly we find ourselves in a room and say, "Why did I just come into this room?" You know, people get very frightened that that might be Alzheimer's, but most of the time, it's actually age-related cognitive decline, and that's because... most people in middle-age are probably in the same job or career that they've had. They might be living in the same town. They might even have the same spouse, if they're lucky – or unlucky – and so on.

So there is not nearly the novelty and demand placed on the brain that we had when we were in high school or university and doing a final exam, okay?

The brain needs to maintain itself, just like the heart. You know, to maintain your heart, you want to do some interval training, or you really want to work up a sweat and challenge it from time to time. Walking is fantastic, but to really get into top shape, you've got to do some exertion.

And the same goes for the brain. You can't spend a lifetime replaying skills you've already mastered, or you can't spend 30 years of middle-age replaying mastered skills, and expect to maintain your brain function.

What has been shown persuasively is that people who are, let's say, 70 who have age-related cognitive decline and who do these brain exercises can start to function the way they did when there were 60 or younger, maybe even 55, maybe even younger, in some cases, and that it generalizes.

So something like Brain HQ is definitely very helpful for maintaining brain function. And it's just so important that you investigate the research backing – not of brain exercises as a category, but of the specific ones you're committing to, because you're putting a lot of time into it.

Now, as for the issue of Alzheimer's, there was a poster [a brief preview, typically at a conference, of not-yet-published research]. The study isn't yet published of using it. They re-analyze that NIH data that I spoke about, and they found that there was a decreased onset. It hasn't gone through the full peer review process. But it was done by the same team that did a ten-year-plus study of brain exercises.

So I don't want to say that brain exercises are part of the package for Alzheimer's based on science. I think, based on prudence, if one was addressing the cellular health the way Dr. Bredesen does, that it does make sense to have that as part of a package.

But my guess is that we're going to see the following very soon: that because there are different kinds, or different pathways to Alzheimer's, it may be helpful for some patients if the general cellular health is being addressed, but maybe not for others.

PEGGY: Well, you make this point again and again in the book: No two brains are the same, no two experiences. And the therapy that works is really individually tailored. So trial and error is probably part of it.

Can you give us just a quick tour? Because I know we have to wrap up now, just a sense of some of the other possibilities? We've got sound, and light, and cognitive exercise. You mentioned the tongue, the tongue as a road into the brain...

DR DOIDGE: Sure.

PEGGY: And maybe some other ones in your book. You talk about cranial stimulation, neuro-feedback. Could you just give us a quick overview of some other interventions?

DR DOIDGE: As I said, I've definitely seen patients get better on tongue simulation. And – again – it doesn't work for everybody all the time, but it was kind of discovered by accident. It involves a lab that I've followed since 2003, and the work of Dr. Paul Bach-y-Rita, who was originally trying to develop a prosthetic device for people who had balance problems.

Balance problems are very common. There was, for instance, a woman, a patient I got to know named Cheryl Scholz. She was prescribed an antibiotic after a hysterectomy that damaged her inner ear, and she completely lost her balance.

So the idea of this device was a plastic strip about the size of a piece of chewing gum that had, I think, 144 little electrical stimulators on it. She'd put it on her tongue, and it would be fixed up to a small computer and to a hat with an accelerometer, which is kind of like a gyroscope. It tells you where you are in space.

She'd lean forward, and because she had no input for balance from her ears, she would feel the electrical stimulation on her tongue, kind of like roll forward. It felt like champagne bubbles. The "champagne bubbles" would roll forward, telling her she was in the forward position. You go to the side; the champagne bubbles go to the side.

Anyway, to make a long story short, that worked magnificently well. But she also found after she took the hat off that the ability to orient in space even without the device would last for a few seconds.

And so she kept using it, and that residual period of normal orientation lasted longer, and longer, and longer. This is a woman who'd lost 97.5% of her ability to orient in space. Eventually, she didn't even need the hat.

A lot of us were thinking about, "What is happening to this woman?" And one of the things was that her brain was developing new pathways or new connections in that 2.5% of her orientation ability that was left, that was taking over her balance function.

So the next thing that happened is the lab said, "Well let's see... Let's do an advertisement for people with balance problems."

Cheryl had a unique condition, a very rare balance condition. So people with balance problems came to the lab, and they put this device on. People with Parkinson's have balance problems. People with stroke have balance problems. People with MS have balance problems. TBI [traumatic brain injury] patients have balance problems. There are a lot of conditions with balance problems.

Their balance improved – but something else happened that was never anticipated. People with Parkinson's felt less rigid. Huh! That wasn't supposed to happen. Mood often goes in Parkinson's. Their mood improved. Same with stroke. People with stroke came in; their balance improved, but maybe their coordination improved.

This didn't make any sense. The researchers were working on a model that was just addressing balance issues. And then someone in the lab figured out that maybe it's the electrical stimulation on the tongue, which is going directly to the brain stem, which is having a generalized resetting effect on what I would call a noisy brain in the brain stem.

So now it's being studied for TBI and other things. I said it was an accidental discovery. You know, we think about what I call consumer science. The president says, "Let's get a man on the moon."

PEGGY: Man on the moon.

DR DOIDGE: Man on the moon. Or let's solve the AIDS problem. Those are two brilliant examples of what I would call consumer science. But that's not the way most science works most of the time.

PEGGY: Right.

DR DOIDGE: Most of the time, we don't understand something, but the scientist is very well-educated, and something happens that's not supposed to happen. And then the alert scientist says, "Obviously my knowledge is very limited. I have to rethink things based on this thing." So you repeat it to make sure it's a real phenomenon, and then you start thinking.

What they realized was that there were many things that were happening in that brain stem area that were being addressed by this technique. And now it's being studied for a number of things, particularly MS, stroke. It's been used at times for Parkinson's and helped some people, and for traumatic brain injury.

So that's a great way to noninvasively sculpt the brain and make use of its plasticity, using a kind of energy-based intervention.

Now, I've mentioned neuro-feedback a few times. Neuro-feedback's been around a long time. The problem with neuro-feedback was that people were making all sorts of claims that didn't make sense to people who had the model of the brain as a machine.

Basically what happens is this: Neuro-feedback in the typical delivery system now would involve having some kind of EEG, a partial EEG feeding signals into a computer, and then to a computer interface.

And neuro-feedback is an evidence-based treatment for certain kinds of epilepsy and ADD. What that means is you train your brain, and then you don't need to take medication – period – if you've got that kind of ADD.

For so many kids with ADD, the teacher says, "Johnny, are you listening, or are you asleep?" And actually, part of Johnny's brain is asleep. That's what's happening. In a lot of kids with ADD there are brain waves that most of us, as adults or teenagers, have as we're falling to sleep. These waves have a much higher representation in Johnny's brain. There are the other brain waves that most of us have when we're in a calm focus that are underrepresented in Johnny's brain.

So what you do is you wire Johnny up, and you find out which brainwaves he's firing at any given time. And even Johnny sometimes will fire those brain waves that have to do with a calm focus, even though he doesn't do it very much.

The computer picks up when the "calm focus" waves are firing, and you might set up a game where there are three boats. And when he's in a state of really calm focus, his boat, the middle boat, surges ahead of the other two boats. And you just tell Johnny this: "Watch the game, and just know that it's really good when your boat wins."

It's set up so that when he has calm-focused waves, he gets a feedback signal: "That's good. Keep doing that. Keep doing that." And when he has fewer of the sleep waves, or sleep-like waves, his boat surges even farther.

Now, it's remarkable, but so much of what we do is unconscious. But all you have to do is just tell Johnny, "It's good when your boat wins," and over time, maybe typically 40 training sessions, what will happen is that he will learn how to shift himself into calm focus when he has to, and not be sleepy in class.

And this is without medication, so it's a spectacular treatment. It's underutilized. And that's just one use or application for neuro-feedback.

It's been helpful in some kinds of epilepsy. It's also been used in some learning disorders. Sometimes in a person two parts of the brain that should be talking to each other are not. So what you can do is you can set the game up so that on the rare instances when they do accidentally shake hands, the boat goes ahead. And you train that over 40 to 60 sessions, and now you can get two parts of the brain talking that, for whatever reason, weren't talking before the therapy.

There are many potential uses of neuro-feedback. And again, it's noninvasive. And it's not propping up a failing system. It's training the brain to do what it ought to have done originally.

PEGGY: So Dr. Doidge, I want to thank you so much for sharing your really unique insights with us today. We've learned how, without taking medication, we can deploy forms of energy like light and sound and doing computer programs, and putting electrical impulses through our tongue – who would've thought of that? – to see improvements in so many conditions that we consider hopeless, like severe learning disorders, and neurodegenerative diseases which don't seem to have any other kind of answer, and strokes – some of the other things that you mentioned today. This is really rich, new information for us. Thank you so much.

And thank you for watching. I hope you were as excited as I was to learn about these really new approaches that have the potential to heal such difficult and challenging conditions. I hope you found it of value. Thank you for watching.

Interview with Dr. Sherri Caplan, M.D.

PEGGY SARLIN: Hello, I'm Peggy Sarlin, and today I'm in Toronto, Canada, where I have the pleasure of speaking with Dr. Sherri Caplan, who's the Founder and the Medical Director of VitalityMD, which is a really unique, one-stop shop for a full spectrum of medical services.

Dr. Caplan has a background in family medicine, but she's also board-certified and a fellow in Antiaging and Regenerative Medicine, and Metabolic and Nutritional Medicine. So she has a very rich background, and a lot of expertise in how hormones, genetics, and environment can have an impact on your brain health.

I also had, really, the great pleasure today of speaking with several of Dr. Caplan's patients, and they shared with me the stories of their journey to better brain health with the help of Dr. Caplan. Now, I'm about to discuss those stories with Dr. Caplan so you can hear and learn from them how to improve your journey to better brain health. I think you're going to learn a lot today.

So welcome, Dr. Caplan.

DR CAPLAN: Thank you for inviting me.

PEGGY: You started out as a family practitioner. You were delivering babies. You had a whole good thing going on there. And then you changed direction, and you became a functional medicine specialist, and that's very dramatic change. What happened? Why did you change?

DR CAPLAN: Well, I think a lot of people start learning about Functional Medicine, or Integrative Medicine, when they start having their own problems. And for me, I started having a lot of perimenopausal symptoms, but not the typical ones, like hot flashes, and vaginal dryness, and stuff like that.

But my symptoms were more about my brain health, like I found my memory wasn't as good as it used to be. I was brilliant. I would learn something once – teach it, do it, right? And then it was sort of like, "Oh, yeah, I kind of remember something." And I'd have to start writing things down, and my energy kind of shifted, and then I started gaining weight, and then it was like, "What's going on?"

And then I guess that tied to my patients sort of all having come in in their 40s, also complaining about weight gain, and I used to tell them, "Oh, you're not eating right, or exercising right." But for me, I was eating right, and I was exercising. So then my thought was, "Ah! It must be hormones."

So I became very interested in that, and I started learning about functional medicine, which looks at the root cause of problems, as opposed to recommending a pill for every ill, and then I started sort of practicing that philosophy with my patients.

And what I really noticed was a shift in their health and wellbeing. And then it was like, "Oh, I'm onto something." It's like the veil was taken off. It was like, "Oh, my gosh, I can't get enough," and I wanted to learn more, and more, and more.

PEGGY: Well, I had the pleasure of speaking with some of your patients, and their stories are instructive, I think, to help other people who are struggling with different health issues. Because these issues tend to be complex, not just one thing, and you're helping them in multiple ways. So let's start talking about some of your patients.

CUT TO: Leslie, a patient

LESLIE: I was struggling. I was really suffering. I was experiencing a lot of chronic pain, a lot of fatigue. I was also in the throes of perimenopause. So along with all of those other sorts of side effects, I was having a lot of mood swings, weight gain, things that I sort of hadn't struggled with before, and they were all kind of new, and not so exciting.

So cognitively, there were big changes as well. There was a significant memory loss. There was a definite lack of focus, to the point where I thought perhaps I had ADHD. There was a definite sort of drop in just having my faculties about me, and being able to find a word, or consider something that I had done in the past that was familiar. So there was a lot of forgetfulness.

CUT TO: Peggy and Dr. Caplan

PEGGY: Let's talk about Leslie. When she came in, she had fibromyalgia. What was her medical condition when she came to see you?

DR CAPLAN: She had like a lot of different things. She had fibromyalgia. She had some mood, some PMS. She was also perimenopausal. She had a lot of gut health issues.

So we needed to work on all of those things, because each one can contribute to weight gain. Having gut inflammation not only can cause brain inflammation and affect mood, but it also contributes to weight.

And also, again, she was deficient on certain nutrients. She was also vegan for a very long time, and vegans may not be getting enough protein. B12's really important. Carnitine's really important. So again, we wanted to replace all those nutrients.

And then there's a whole genetic piece involved in weight. There are certain things that I can pick out by a patient's history to guess that they might be genetically predisposed.

PEGGY: Like what? What would be a red flag for you?

DR CAPLAN: Well, certain things in their history. People who may have fibromyalgia, ADD, autism, migraine sufferers, dizziness and vertigo seem to have a genetic issue with B12, and they might be low on that vitamin. Plus, she was vegan, so you have to be really meticulous on replacing B12.

PEGGY: So let's just stop there for a minute. Genetically, what... Genetically, you can't absorb B12? What's the genetic connection with how you process B12?

DR CAPLAN: There are different genetic snips that relate to B12, so it's not just one. So one is the absorption of B12. The other one may be the ability of the receptor to bring whatever's in the serum into the cells. So there are different deficiencies or genetics that predispose you. Some people may actually have a normal blood level, but actually still might be deficient intracellularly. So we look at that.

PEGGY: So let's talk about it in relationship to Leslie. Tell me, your diagnosis – she came in with these symptoms. You told her to do XYZ, and how is she now?

DR CAPLAN: So for her, we sort of looked at her diet and replaced deficient nutrients. We balanced her hormones, because she was also perimenopausal and had bad PMS.

And then we attacked gut health, and we had her follow a very specific diet in conjunction with some IV therapy. That sort of gave her back the amino acids that she needed as building blocks, but improved her detox pathways.

She was someone who was generally healthy to begin with. She was a big yoga person and exercised tons, but still was gaining weight. When she started doing our protocol, she lost a significant amount of weight, and then, in the process, felt significantly better.

CUT TO:

LESLIE: So I spoke to Dr. Caplan about this. I was very concerned, and she put me on a rotation of supplements that were incredibly helpful for cognitive health. On top of that, I also began doing IV therapy weekly at the clinic, and that was incredible for me. It helped me with pain management from the fibro. It helped with the cognitive functioning incredibly.

We talked a lot about alternative healing, like infrared saunas, continuing a meditation practice, managing stress in my life... all kinds of sort of healing therapies, and then continuing the lifestyle of good health. She rebalanced my diet in such a way that I was still able to eat a very sort of healthful type of nutritional lifestyle, but just re-proportioning my foods on my plate for me.

So we sort of released some of those things, brought in more protein, more greens, more color, and instead of struggling with the weight loss, it just fell right off, like that, yeah.

PEGGY: Tell us about that. How do you feel that you handled that experience with this, your new health regimen?

LESLIE: Well, I just had half my lung removed two weeks ago, so I recovered...

PEGGY: You're beautiful!

LESLIE: ...really quickly.

PEGGY: Two weeks ago?

LESLIE: Mm hm. So I think because I positioned myself in such a way that I set myself up in a really healthy way before my surgery, it really helped with my recovery, yes.

PEGGY: You're inspiring everybody who's listening to you right now.

LESLIE: Thank you.

PEGGY: You're offering us all a lot of inspiration.

LESLIE: Thank you. Thank you, thank you.

CUT TO: Peggy and Dr. Caplan

PEGGY: Okay, so Leslie now feels good, and let's talk about Mary, whom I had the pleasure of meeting. Mary came to you. She had a whole complicated medical history. There are a lot of things... tell us what, from your perspective. You took her history. What seemed relevant, and what were the symptoms that you were looking for?

DR CAPLAN: Mary had a few things going on, and one was a concussion. And I think we need to talk a little bit of concussion...

CUT TO: Mary, a patient

MARY: Well, it started about ten years ago, where I was diagnosed with Hashimoto's, and I was monitored with medication with that, and that seemed to control it. And then, about five years ago, I sustained a bad concussion riding horses.

PEGGY: Oh.

MARY: And I recovered from that. It took about six months.

And then following that, about a year later, I got a bad viral flu infection with a high fever, and then after that, probably about a week after that, I started having heart palpitations, massive anxiety, inability to sleep, inability to eat. And I went to my doctor saying, "You know something, this flu's caused it, because I didn't feel that way before."

And she said, "No, no, no. You're just an anxious person. Here, have some Prozac." So she gave me a half dose. I didn't want it. She said, "Here, just try a half dose. You'll feel much better."

PEGGY: Wow.

MARY: So I went home, thinking, "Okay, I must be crazy," because it definitely seemed to be linked to this flu bug I had. But clearly, I'm not a doctor, so I followed her orders and took the Prozac. And after about three weeks, I didn't feel any better. In fact, I felt worse. So I went back to her, and she put me on a full dose of Prozac.

So I went home on the full dose, and another three weeks went by, and by this time I've lost about 12 pounds, and I can't ride. I can't – I have three boys. I couldn't sleep. It was challenging to parent them, and my poor husband just could – it was as if I transformed from this functional person into a wreck.

So I talked to a friend in the States who's a functional doctor, and she suggested that possibly it's my thyroid, and that I needed to find a doctor up here who could look at the big picture.

So luckily I found Dr. Caplan, who I came to a total mess, in tears. I couldn't even speak, because I just had these waves of anxiety and heart palpitations – basically, the feeling you get right after you almost have a car crash.

CUT TO: Peggy and Dr. Caplan

PEGGY: So Mary had these three factors that we know of: the thyroid, the concussion and the virus.

DR CAPLAN: What I've learned with the head concussion is that two big things actually happen. One is that you have the initial injury, and you have inflammation. But it actually sets off another cascade of cytokines and other inflammatory markers that can be ongoing, not just initially, but actually for years. And unless you stop that inflammation, you can actually cause damage.

And then the other thing that happens is that with the trauma, you can actually have what's called axonal injury, where the nerves or the axons are damaged, and the communication links between different parts of the brain aren't working. They may not be totally severed, but that feedback is not working, or the sensor is off.

And so basically, the thyroid may not work optimally, or the person's testosterone or other hormones may be off, and by the way there's plenty of literature that shows that low testosterone causes depression. Low DHEA can cause depression. Low thyroid can cause depression.

So when patients have a head injury, I, again, want to look at their bloodwork for inflammatory markers. I want to look at hormonal balance. You know, where are they fitting in the range? Are they at the low end? Is it outside the range? Where are they? And I want to optimize those things.

And then also I want to reduce the inflammation, so I'll use a lot of supplements to reduce inflammation in the brain – to stop that ongoing message that says there's damage.

And what's really neat is that inflammation can cause more hormonal disruption as well. Why? Well, we now know that neurons actually have the ability to make hormones themselves. So actually, neurons can make estrogen, progesterone, testosterone, DHEA, and pregnenolone. We also know that our hormones help with repair and regeneration.

So in an environment where there's inflammation, you lose that ability to make those hormones. And then, if that person also happens to be perimenopausal or menopausal, where they're losing those hormones, or in men, where they go through andropause, and they're low on testosterone, not only are you losing your peripheral hormones that have an effect on the brain, but you've also lost the neurosteroids, or those hormones that are being produced in the brain. So you're losing that capacity for repair and regeneration.

PEGGY: So the brain itself makes hormones.

DR CAPLAN: Correct.

PEGGY: And most of us don't think if...

DR CAPLAN: But only if there's no inflammation.

PEGGY: Only if there's no inflammation. But when everything's healthy, and you don't have the inflammation, you've got a nice hormone factory going on in the brain.

DR CAPLAN: Correct. And each hormone has a different effect. For example, estrogen basically helps protect the brain against Alzheimer's, but it actually relates to two neurotransmitters. One is acetylcholine, which essentially is your concentration and your memory, and then the other one is serotonin, which is your happy hormone.

So again, in a concussion, if you're losing your estrogen, then your memory and your mood can be off, and that will actually happen perimenopausally, as well. So it sort of becomes a double whammy if the person's in perimenopause, and has a head injury.

And then progesterone binds to the GABA receptors, which function as your natural tranquilizer and sleep aid. So somebody who has head injury and loses their progesterone, or again, is in perimenopause, then they lose their natural tranquilizer and sleep aid, and what are they going to present to their doctor? "I'm not sleeping. I'm feeling anxious." And what's the regular doctor going to do? "Oh, here's your antidepressant or sleeping pill."

PEGGY: Yeah, or both.

DR CAPLAN: Or both.

CUT TO: Mary

MARY: So Dr. Caplan, in her capable hands, looked at the big picture. She looked at my bloodwork. We looked at my diet. We looked at my mental health, my exercise program.

She looked at everything, which was fantastic, and one of the things she found was that my reverse T-3 was sky high, so we changed my thyroid medication. And I was perimenopausal, so I was on some bioidentical hormones, but she changed that up. And diet-wise, I went gluten-free, dairy-free, sugar-free – basically, paleo.

She saved my life. It was amazing, having the support, and having a doctor who would take the time – not take three minutes, look at you, say, "Here's some drugs. See you next week," or, you know, "Come back in a month, and let me know."

So having the support of a doctor who was interested in exploring, and would listen to me. So when I said, "You know, I think maybe I had this flu bug. Maybe it could be that," she didn't dismiss anything that I had to say.

CUT TO: Peggy and Rob, a patient

PEGGY: Okay, so you had a concussion, and then you had another concussion, and that's when things kind of spiraled out of control.

ROB: Yeah, so you know, for a good three, or four, or five years, I was trying all sorts of different things, spending money in all sorts of different directions. And everybody would just say, "Hey, I've got what it is. You know, you go ahead, and this is what it's going to be, and it's going to take two months," and nothing would happen.

Until finally I saw Dr. Caplan, and everything that she was talking about was more like there was these biomarkers. It was like, "Let's get your blood work done, and let's see what it shows, and then let's make a decision based on that."

Everybody else that I talked to would say something like, "Oh, what are your symptoms? Okay, well then, you know, maybe you should do this for your symptoms. Maybe you should slow down, Rob. Maybe that's what it is."

But with Dr. Caplan it was, "Let's take a look at his blood results. Let's see where the inefficiencies are, and then we can go through a supplement program. We can talk about diet. We can talk about reducing inflammation."

You know, there was a very high marker that I had in the blood work. And again, this – I think it was called the CRP level.

PEGGY: Yeah, it is.

ROB: But it was something to sort of detect inflammation that most people get tested, maybe males, after 50. It's something to do with cardiovascular disease, and mine was through the roof – like ten times where it should be. And so that was one of the markers. It was like, "We need to reduce your inflammation." So she talked about diet.

I had gone to this head injury clinic for three or four years. They never once talked to me about taking fish oil, or talked about reducing sugars, and processed foods, and food high in fats, or taking these supplements – or the word inflammation did not even come up.

And this was one meeting that I just came here, and I was like, "Wow, I can't believe that I've been going to all these different people, and not one person said, 'Hey, maybe we should take a look at some blood work. Maybe that's like a biomarker that we can use to get you in the right direction,'" kind of thing, right?

PEGGY: This is very important stuff. A lot of people have head injuries. You know, it's very, very common, so you're doing something valuable by sharing this.

ROB: Gradually over time, it got me back. And it gave me some focus. It was like, "Okay, this inflammation is the key here. That's what I've got to reduce."

My diet changed completely, cutting out gluten, and making sure there were no sugars, and chocolates, and, you know, putting lots of avocados in my diet and coconut oil, and all sorts of different stuff like that, right? Curcumin, and, like, turmeric – all this kind of stuff that she was telling me about, and she does a ton of research.

CUT TO: Peggy and Dr. Caplan

DR CAPLAN: So back to the head injury and the inflammation. We actually know that certain people are genetically predisposed, that when they have a head injury, they have a higher likelihood of sequela. So on...

PEGGY: What's sequela?

DR CAPLAN: Outcomes, like problems. So you know, one person can hit their head and have no problems whatsoever, and then the next person hits their head with the same intensity, and all of a sudden they have more cognitive dysfunction, or they're having imbalances and whatnot.

And again, looking at certain genetic snips, which relate to either B12, or their Vitamin D receptor, or to some other ones that actually can tell us who's more likely to have a problem after a head injury.

And wouldn't it be neat if we actually could test all our young folks before they start doing competitive sports, and identify all those who are at risk, and make sure that they're on omega 3 oil, B vitamins, and vitamin D? Or if we don't want to spend the money on the genetics, then at least recommend that everybody who's playing contact sports or is likely to hit their head should be on those three basic nutrients, because it will prevent a problem if they have an injury.

PEGGY: The three basic nutrients, just to – once again, these are so important for controlling inflammation...

DR CAPLAN: And helping those genetic predispositions. So those were the B vitamins...

PEGGY: The B vitamins.

DR CAPLAN: Specifically, B12 and B6, and actually, folic acid, while we're at it, and then omega...

PEGGY: Omega.

DR CAPLAN: ...and making sure your vitamin D is at an optimal level, because everybody's genetically different, and we have different genetic snips that make our absorption or utilization of vitamin D different. So actually, it is important to have your vitamin D level checked, because one person can get away with 1,000 units a day, and somebody might need 8,000 to get that same blood level.

PEGGY: Well, one of the things you and I have talked about is the importance of growth hormone, in terms of stimulating the birth of new brain cells. Tell us how that might be effective, and what can we do for that?

DR CAPLAN: When we have a full complement of our hormones, where we have enough estrogen, progesterone, testosterone, DHEA, pregnenolone, and have low cortisol, low insulin, you know, that helps with the repair and regeneration, and that we have optimal growth hormone levels.

So there are certain things that, again, you can do that help stimulate growth hormone naturally. And then there are certain secretagogues, meaning a mixture of certain things that will raise growth hormone naturally. The presence of these factors increases the secretion of growth hormone.

I will often use something called secretropin in my practice for...

PEGGY: Let's stop and spell that for everybody, because we haven't come upon that word before. It's a new option for us.

DR CAPLAN: Right, so secretropin is S-E-C-R-E-T-R-O-P-I-N.

PEGGY: Secretropin.

DR CAPLAN: ...-tropin, correct. So it's...

PEGGY: Secret, as in – not as in secret. It's secret, as in, it's being secreted.

DR CAPLAN: Correct.

PEGGY: Okay.

DR CAPLAN: So it increases the secretion.

PEGGY: Okay, the secretion. Okay.

DR CAPLAN: Yes, so it's called secretropin.

PEGGY: And this is a prescription drug?

DR CAPLAN: Well, it's an amino acid mix that you need a healthcare provider to recommend in order to get it. So in that way, it's kind of like a prescription, whereas this drug actually was created in the States for veterans to help with their traumatic brain injury. And then in the States, they now have Dynatropin that is available without a recommendation of either a medical doctor, or a naturopathic doctor, so...

PEGGY: You can just go to a health food store, or online, and buy Dynatropin?

DR CAPLAN: Correct.

PEGGY: And what's Dynatropin? It sounds like it's the fountain of youth.

DR CAPLAN: Well, essentially, it's something that is great. It helps people who have traumatic brain injury. It helps with their focus, and it helps stimulate growth hormone that, again, helps with that repair and regeneration. Now again, it's not just one thing, it's never one thing that's the answer.

PEGGY: It's not one thing.

DR CAPLAN: It's really that multifactorial thing. So it's eating right, improving your gut health, exercising, de-stressing, meditating, replacing those deficient nutrients, optimizing your hormones. It's that whole protocol that really makes the difference. So it's sort of a similar story with some different pieces to it.

PEGGY: Well, the Dynatropin is going to help. We want our hippocampus to be creating new brain cells, right? We always want to be regenerating, and having our brain creating new cells. But if things go ideally, and we're doing these other wonderful lifestyle things, is it reasonable to think that Dynatropin is going to stimulate growth hormone, which is then going to stimulate new cells?

DR CAPLAN: Well, yes. I think, again, it's one of those pieces.

We actually can grow new neurons, for sure. And basically, there's many things that can do that. Exercise is one of those things. Eating fruits and vegetables, colorful, rainbow-colored produce, reducing inflammation, having curcumin, playing a musical instrument, learning something new. All of these things help with new neurons. So again, yes, we want to do things to create new nerves, and then we want to stop those bad habits that actually kill them.

PEGGY: We're going to have to wrap up soon, but in speaking to your patients, it was interesting that certain things happened to them that seemed to precipitate things getting worse, and their doctors ignored them.

One of them, Rob, had suffered two serious concussions. He noticed that when he went on an airplane, when he flew, his condition deteriorated. His doctor wasn't terribly interested in that, but what can you tell us about flying? What should we know?

DR CAPLAN: Actually, there's some data to show that when we fly, we get inflamed. There are case reports of ulcerative colitis getting worse, and Crohn's getting worse after someone flies. So there is this inflammation that goes on.

Certain people, based on their genetics, may make more reactive oxygen species – that's ROS, is the abbreviation – and flying may exacerbate it. And what I actually tell people to do in that case is take antioxidants right before they fly.

PEGGY: What should they take?

DR CAPLAN: Good things like vitamin C, N-acetylcysteine, or NAC, is the abbreviation.

PEGGY: NAC, yeah.

DR CAPLAN: You can take glutathione, curcumin, high-dose omega. Any of those things would be a good thing to take pre-flight. And what they'll usually find is they get less leg swelling, they feel less bloated. And those migraines can flare with the barometric pressure. The guts can get irritated. So hopefully, all of those supplements may help prevent that from happening.

PEGGY: That's very good knowledge for all of us, that flying in a plane, which a lot of us do, can have an effect on our brain, and we can preempt that problem by taking antioxidants. Who knew? Not a common piece of knowledge.

The other issue – Mary talked about a virus. The virus precipitated... It doesn't just come and go away. It precipitated other things happening. And once again, her doctor wasn't interested in that.

So maybe the piece of this I want to ask you is, I'm getting the theme, talking to your patients, that their bodies are telling them things. The doctors aren't listening, but their bodies are trying to signal to them that something's wrong. So can you tell us about that?

DR CAPLAN: Yes. Through functional medicine, one of the things we tend to ask is, "Has there been a major life change, or a major stress?" And one of those stresses could be a viral illness, a bacterial illness... you know, something that's significant. Because all of those things cause inflammation, and that can start a cascade, a downward turn.

And also, with regard to autoimmunity, what we know is there's something called molecular mimicry. So what does that mean?

Let's say you get a virus. You produce antibodies against that virus, and then that antibody that you created cross-reacts with your own tissue. So depending on what that is, you can get rheumatoid arthritis, or you might get Reiter's syndrome, or thyroiditis, or something else.

So there is that relationship, and so, yes, it's kind of neat, but if you go back, a lot of people say, "Oh, I had a case of mono, and ever since I had mono, I'm not the same. I have brain fog. My energy's down," and all these other things.

PEGGY: Some people say that after surgery with the anesthesia, they don't feel their brain is the same.

DR CAPLAN: Well, again, it's a toxin. We accumulate those toxins, and if you don't improve that detox pathway, some people will accumulate more. And yes, it all has an effect.

PEGGY: So we're hearing a lot today about inflammation as a common problem; about hormonal changes happening in midlife; more women get Alzheimer's than men, and perhaps, this is a piece of that puzzle, this hormonal mid-life change.

We're learning about a toxic load, and the need to detox through exercise and other means in order to release the toxins from our brain. These are common themes. We hear different stories, but we keep coming back to these themes.

So we've learned a lot today. What do you want us to leave with, in terms of our marching orders, to keeping our brains healthy?

DR CAPLAN: I think it's what I tell my patients every day: learn to eat better – like, don't eat processed foods. Go back to the way we were supposed to eat, things like protein, fruits and vegetables. Eat all colors of the rainbow.

Get sufficient omega-3. De-stress, whatever way you choose – exercise, meditation, connecting with people. I mean, we don't see that happening as much anymore. Everybody's, like, busy texting on their phones or whatnot.

And balancing your hormones, if appropriate, and if you're past a certain age and you're looking at estrogen and progesterone, you still need to balance your thyroid, and your cortisol levels, and your leptin levels...

You know, there's so many other pieces, and really replacing those deficient nutrients. And it's really important to look at the data and see what's there. And it's not good enough to be in the low normal. You want to be optimal.

PEGGY: You want to be optimal. We all want to be optimal. That's a good note to end on...

So thank you, Dr. Caplan, for sharing your expertise with us, and for telling us about your clinic here, where so many services are available, and of course, for inviting your patients to come and get personal, and tell their stories and their journeys to healing. So I wish you good health, and all your patients that are lucky enough to work with you. May they all have good health, and thank you so much.

DR CAPLAN: Well, thank you.

PEGGY: And thank you for watching. I hope you learned from the real-life stories of Dr. Caplan's patients. I hope you learned useful information for your real-life story, and your journey to healing. Thank you.

Interview with Jacob Teitelbaum, M.D.

PEGGY: Hello, I'm Peggy Sarlin, and today I'm speaking with Dr. Jacob Teitelbaum in Laguna Beach, California. Dr. Teitelbaum is going to tell us five ways to tune up your brain and turn on your memory.

Dr. Teitelbaum is a board certified internist. He's a nationally recognized expert in integrative medicine. He is the creator of the smart phone app, "Cures A-Z," and he's one of my most favorite knowledgeable people to go to for information about the brain. So welcome, Dr. Teitelbaum.

DR TEITELBAUM: Peggy, awesome to be with you. And today we're going to teach people that 80 really is the new 50.

PEGGY: 80 is the new 50.

DR TEITELBAUM: But here's the thing: Can you imagine if you had a car with 80,000 miles on it, and you had never once had a tune-up? That car would run like a real clunker. But then you go give it a tune-up, and suddenly it sounds like a new car. My car has over 80,000 miles on it. It runs like a new car because I give it a tune-up every so often.

PEGGY: You give it a tune up. Tuning up our brain is within our power if we know what to do.

DR TEITELBAUM: And tuning up our whole body, in fact. Why not get everything right, and let your brain get better with it? People find they feel dramatically better. Now, some people say, "But I go to my doctor every year for a checkup."

PEGGY: Right. A checkup is not a tune-up.

DR TEITELBAUM: No. A checkup is where you go in to see if you have "it" yet, "it" being some very expensive-to-treat disease. But when's the last time you went in that the doctor actually did anything to make you feel better and optimize your function? For most of you, the answer is "never."

PEGGY: Never.

DR TEITELBAUM: So we're going to teach you five tips for tuning up your body, and a simple way you can do it on your own. In fact, let me give people a resource they can consult.

On the website, www.endfatigue.com...

PEGGY: www.endfatigue.com, Dr. Teitelbaum's website.

DR TEITELBAUM: You'll see a free energy analysis program. You go on the website; you do a quiz. You can even plug in the pertinent lab tests if you want, if you have them, and it'll tell you which ones would be helpful, but they're not critical. You don't have to have the labs to do this. It'll analyze all of that.

I actually hold a U.S. patent for computerized doctor that we developed for people with fibromyalgia and chronic fatigue syndrome, because our studies showed that it was treatable, but it's complex to treat.

The free energy analysis program will analyze all this, optimize your energy production, and tell you, "Here's what's going on that's draining your energy. Here's what you need for a tune-up."

And most of these things you can do on your own.

PEGGY: OK, this is interesting because you keep coming back to the concept of energy, increasing energy. When you get a little bit older, a very common complaint is senior moments, forgetfulness, a sluggish brain, brain fog. These are all kind of symptoms of low cognitive energy. Is that right?

DR TEITELBAUM: There is not enough energy in the brain for the brain to function properly.

PEGGY: So if we tune up the brain, we're going to increase cognitive energy. Our brain's just going to be – what is the expression – they're going to be firing more? They're going to be creating...?

DR TEITELBAUM: You're going to have neurotransmitters that are working. The synapses are going to be much more efficient, and all of the chemical reactions actually can go back to what they were when you were in your 30's and 40's.

Now, let me offer a couple quick things, though, Peggy, for people. 1) You know how sometimes you go into a room and you forget what you went in for, or you're looking for your keys and you forget where you left the keys. And when you were 20, if that happened you didn't think twice about it. Like, who cares?

But it's different when you're 50, and 60, and 70, and all your friends are talking about Alzheimer's and worried about this...

Now, Alzheimer's is not when you forget where you left the keys. Alzheimer's is when you forget how to use the keys.

PEGGY: Oh, that's much farther down the road.

DR TEITELBAUM: So don't drive yourself nuts if you're just having a normal, day-to-day kind of a thing, because you've had that all your life.

PEGGY: But let's go back to the tune-up idea. If we're seeing increasing frequency, and incidents where you say, "I just don't remember. I can't find my glasses. Where's my wallet?" – if this is happening more and more, this seems to be a symptom, then you need a tune-up.

DR TEITELBAUM: ...of low energy in the brain.

PEGGY: You have low brain energy and you need to get your neurotransmitters talking to the synapses, and all this kind of thing.

DR TEITELBAUM: You've got to give your brain a tune-up.

PEGGY: You've got to tune up. All right. How are we going to tune up our brain? Help me tune up my brain.

DR TEITELBAUM: What our research shows is that to optimize energy you optimize with what you call the "SHINE Protocol."

PEGGY: This is your own proprietary protocol.

DR TEITELBAUM: Well, it's funny, because I tend to be a bit of a medical curmudgeon. I don't like it when medical ideas are patented. So we actually patented the SHINE Protocol, and then donated the patent into the public domain so anybody can use it, and nobody else can try to patent it and make it their property – so people can use that.

PEGGY: We like that. Okay, so you developed this. We'll do it that way.

DR TEITELBAUM: And it's not proprietary. Anybody can use it. Yes, I developed it.

PEGGY: You developed it.

DR TEITELBAUM: So "S" is for sleep.

PEGGY: Sleep.

DR TEITELBAUM: You want to optimize sleep and get your eight hours sleep a night. The average night's sleep in the United States used to be nine hours a night until lightbulbs, 135 years ago. Now we're down to 6 ½, and that's nowhere near enough to recharge the brain chemicals, the neurotransmitters and other things that your brain needs to function.

So you're using the [brain energy] today, and at nighttime your body is recharging the battery. But if you're losing 30% of your sleep, that's not happening.

PEGGY: You're right. You're going to get that sluggish brain and that forgetfulness because hormones need to be created during sleep that aren't being created. Is this accurate?

DR TEITELBAUM: A lot of your hormones, neurotransmitters, growth hormone... Growth hormone is called "The Fountain of Youth Hormone." It's made during exercise, sex and deep sleep.

PEGGY: All good things.

DR TEITELBAUM: All good things. Now how do you get to sleep without making yourself fuzzy the next day? Well, there's a mix of herbals called the Revitalizing Sleep Formula. It's six herbs, leaves most people sleeping like a puppy. Add a half a milligram of melatonin to it. It doesn't take any more than that.

You may also find a nice, hot Epsom salt bath at bedtime helpful. You take two – especially in the wintertime in the North – you take two cups of Epsom salts, magnesium salts, in a tub of hot water. Soak.

Pour yourself a little bit of wine. I know people are giving you all kinds of grief about that, but if you have four ounces of wine it's fine for bedtime. Even have a little bit of chocolate, even though it has a little theobromine stimulant. Light some candles. Relax. Set yourself up a routine for sleep.

If you find that you're waking up to pee a lot at night, get an herb called "SagaPro."

PEGGY: SagaPro.

DR TEITELBAUM: And that will help with urinary urgency and even –

PEGGY: For men? For women? For everybody?

DR TEITELBAUM: Both. So if you're a woman and you find that you laugh so hard that the tears run down your legs – you know that kind of a thing? – take the SagaPro. If you're waking up all night to pee, take the SagaPro.

PEGGY: SagaPro, okay – that's a good, helpful tip.

DR TEITELBAUM: Yeah. Nice, simple things. So there's all kinds of natural things you can do for sleep. The smell of lavender. Take a little lavender oil, put it on your upper lip, or if you spray it on the pillow, that will help you sleep at night. And none of these things will leave you hung over.

PEGGY: Right. They're not going to have the side effects that you would get from a prescription medication that makes for all kinds of problems down the road.

DR TEITELBAUM: And even over the counter sleep medicines. For example, if you're taking Unisom for sleep, or Benadryl, or any of these kind of things, they can be very helpful for sleep, but they've been shown to increase the risk of Alzheimer's.

PEGGY: Uh oh!

DR TEITELBAUM: And they can worsen memory. So if it's not causing any problems, they're fine for sleep. But if you're feeling fuzzy, that's not the thing to take.

PEGGY: We know we need to, so the very first thing in your SHINE Protocol is sleep, because we need to get into deep sleep where we're going to be creating these neurotransmitters and hormones, and so forth.

Okay, we've done that. Now we're sleeping like a baby, eight hours a night. Now what are we doing? "H"...

DR TEITELBAUM: Optimize hormones. The thyroid, adrenal, and the reproductive hormones.

PEGGY: "H" is for hormones.

DR TEITELBAUM: Right, so take thyroid – the blood test for thyroid will miss the large majority of people who need thyroid hormones. And we can talk about why the normal ranges doctors rely on are absurd. Let me give a quick overview of that.

The normal range is based on two standard deviations from the mean or average. They take 100 people; the 95 in the middle are considered normal, and only the highest and lowest 2½% are defined as abnormal. They are two standard deviations away from the average.

So a normal shoe size would be 5-13, a normal range. That doesn't mean that I can put my size 12 feet in a size 6 shoe and have it be okay.

PEGGY: Right.

DR TEITELBAUM: You have to look at the symptoms and the shoe size, and the overall picture, and then assess. So how do you tell if you need a trial prescription of thyroid hormone? Tired, achy, weight gain, cold intolerant, constipation... these are symptoms of low thyroid function, and you'll need to find a holistic doctor.

PEGGY: So Doctor, you mentioned that this is the kind of study that a holistic doctor can do. You need to find a holistic doctor. You're going to give us some advice how to go about doing that. But why a holistic doctor? I mean, it may be extra time, expense, effort to find such a doctor. Why is it worth it?

DR TEITELBAUM: Well, understand, it was a shock to me in medical school when I realized that virtually everything that I was being taught was, basically, slick advertising on the part of the drug companies, masquerading as science.

If something was expensive and profitable, it didn't matter if it was effective. It didn't matter if it would kill you. They were spending $35 million per drug, per year, advertising it to physicians, another $35 million to the public.

And what I would do – being a geek, I tend to go through the science literature a lot. I would read thousands and thousands of studies, several hours a day, often. And it was a shock when I realized that these studies – and these were ones that were spoon-fed me by the drug companies – were showing all these natural remedies were really effective and helpful. And it was like, why didn't anybody teach me this stuff? And I said, well, probably because it doesn't work.

And I tried it with some folks. People with end-stage heart failure are out living their lives feeling healthy again. All kinds of things, and I was saying to myself, "What?" Then I realized that basically, if it is cheap and not patentable – which means anything natural, because it's not patentable –

PEGGY: Right.

DR TEITELBAUM: – It can't go through the FDA approval process, which is $400-plus million, and therefore the doctors will never hear about it. But the holistic doctors will look at both the standard research and standard medical options, and also these other studies to see all of the things that can help you.

So if you think about it, it's as if your standard doctor only had a hammer in their tool kit, and that's all they had. So if they needed a wrench, they'd still whack you with a hammer, and you'd feel like the nail... where the holistic doctors have the entire tool kit to use, and that can help you get better.

So when your doctor says, "I'm sorry. There's nothing I can do for you," they're right. There's nothing *they* can do.

PEGGY: They can do.

DR TEITELBAUM: It doesn't mean there's nothing that can be done.

PEGGY: And certainly when you're experiencing forgetfulness, confusion, that might be something that you hear from a doctor. "Well, you're getting older. What do you expect? You're a little bit older." But in fact, you can tune up your brain.

DR TEITELBAUM: Yes, there's a whole lot that you can do, and you're not going to do it in the five minutes that the average doctor is allotted. You really need to take the time, and take an hour or two, and get things tuned up properly, and a holistic doctor can spend that time.

PEGGY: Okay, so we're on our SHINE Protocol. We're optimizing our hormones, which a holistic doctor is going to be attuned to know how to do.

DR TEITELBAUM: Exactly. And they know that the blood tests don't say if you need hormones or not. They just tell you where you fall out of 100 people. Are you in the lowest 5 percentiles, 10, 20, 30...?

But to look at symptoms – tired, achy, weight gain, cold intolerant, constipated – a holistic doctor may give you a trial of thyroid hormone unless there's a reason not to.

If you get irritable when hungry, which is basically adrenal fatigue...

PEGGY: Adrenal fatigue.

DR TEITELBAUM: ...low blood sugar...

PEGGY: That's a very common one, isn't it?

DR TEITELBAUM: It's very common. And if you find that you have these feed-me-now-or-I'll-kill-you moments... But it's funny. The media's talking now about being "hangry," and they're actually advertising advice to eat sugared bars for it, and my reaction is, "But that's what causes the problem."

PEGGY: That's not good advice.

DR TEITELBAUM: It's insane. But you can help the adrenals by increasing salt and water. Salt actually is heathy for most people, unless you have heart failure. Even with high blood pressure, salt restriction only lowers blood pressure less than one point. It's a minimal thing.

PEGGY: But salt helps your adrenals.

DR TEITELBAUM: It helps your adrenals. Also, I like a product called "Adrenal Stress End." It's a mix of licorice, Vitamin B5, adrenal gland solution and Vitamin C, and that supports healthy adrenal function. So you can optimize that. You'll know in a couple days of taking it whether you're going to feel better.

Estrogen, testosterone – use the bioidentical forms of these hormones, and at optimized levels. Don't use the synthetics. They're poison.

And also, when it comes to the reproductive hormones – just because the patient is not reproducing anymore doesn't mean your body doesn't need them. Optimize testosterone in men and women, and optimize using bioidentical estrogen and progesterone. You'll find a major difference in how you feel.

PEGGY: Okay, so we've optimized our adrenals, our thyroids, our estrogen, our testosterone. We're feeling good. Now let's keep moving along with your protocol.

DR TEITELBAUM: "I" would be infections.

PEGGY: "I" is the infections.

DR TEITELBAUM: And the infection to treat would be candida. There's no test for candida, or yeast overgrowth. How do you tell you have it? If you have post-nasal drip, clearing your throat a lot... if you have chronic sinusitis or nasal congestion... or if you have irritable bowel syndrome – gas, bloating, diarrhea, or constipation.

PEGGY: Those are very, very common afflictions.

DR TEITELBAUM: Yes, and you'll find when you treat the candida these things go away. And you can look at my app, "Cures A-Z." It's a free app. There's a $2 upgrade. It'll go through how to treat the candida, how to optimize immune function, to rebalance and get a healthy gut function and sinus function.

PEGGY: Well, most people are probably not thinking, "Oh, I feel a little forgetful today. I'm having trouble concentrating. I couldn't remember my neighbor's name. I might have a yeast infection." That's not necessarily a first thought.

DR TEITELBAUM: But again, yeast infection is a drag on the system. It basically puts a hole in your energy bucket, and it's hard to keep the energy up when you have these chronic infections.

PEGGY: So that's a great point, we're going to go to your website, www.endfatigue.com, or get your smart phone app, "Cures A-Z", and you're going to help us understand what we need to do to knock out the candida.

DR TEITELBAUM: And that's the main infection, really.

PEGGY: The most common one is the candida.

DR TEITELBAUM: And then "N" is nutritional support.

PEGGY: Nutritional support.

DR TEITELBAUM: And nutritional support's easy. You want to eat a good, healthy diet overall, but it's okay to have some junk in the diet, too. Diets should be fun.

I'm going to bust a couple myths. Eggs – you hear that they raise cholesterol. They don't. You can eat six eggs a day for six weeks. Study after study after study shows no effect on cholesterol. Salt – if you restrict salt to the government guidelines for salt intake, there's one major benefit: You die younger, and the Social Security system thanks you.

PEGGY: I don't think that's a benefit!

DR TEITELBAUM: Well, the Social Security system thanks you.

PEGGY: For them, not for you.

DR TEITELBAUM: The experts are saying, "Why are we still giving these guidelines for salt restriction? They're absurd." Chocolate. Chocolate is associated with a 40-50% lower risk of heart attack if you eat just a small square each day.

PEGGY: Dark chocolate.

DR TEITELBAUM: It doesn't matter if it's dark chocolate.

PEGGY: Oh, it doesn't matter if it's dark chocolate!

DR TEITELBAUM: A new study, all kinds were beneficial. Now, if you look at the cholesterol-lowering medications in people with no heart disease and high cholesterol, medication only decreases heart attack deaths on the order of about 2%, 2-10%. So eating chocolate is as much as 25 times more likely to prevent a heart attack than taking a statin drug, or taking...

PEGGY: And it's much more fun!

DR TEITELBAUM: Yeah, I'm not a big fan of the statin medications. If you have known heart disease, they're a lifesaver. But to treat a number on a blood test?

PEGGY: No.

DR TEITELBAUM: In my humble opinion. So – simple things.

The American diet has lost over half of the vitamins and minerals in food processing, and that's why we didn't need a multivitamin 500 years ago, but now we desperately need them.

And it's a simple thing to do, because you don't want to take handfuls of pills all day. I recommend one called the "Energy Revitalization System Vitamin Powder." You can find it in most health food stores. You can find it at www.endfatigue.com . Take one-half to one scoop a day. That'll set you back about twenty-five to seventy-five cents a day. It's not expensive.

And some people find that, because of the powerful nutrition and the magnesium and Vitamin C, the supplement powder may cause some loose stools. Most people find they're more regular, and they like it. But if that's a problem, just lower the dose. But if you take the one-half to one scoop of that a day, people are going to find their brain is back.

PEGGY: Their brain is back.

DR TEITELBAUM: And the whole body is back. Their energy is back.

It was funny... I used to live in Annapolis, Maryland, and I was walking down the street one day, and this guy's looking at me from across the street. And I was, like, looking back at him, and he's looking at me... I never saw this guy in my life.

Suddenly he's dashing through traffic across the street, runs up to me, grabs me in a bear hug, lifts me up in the air and says, "You're Dr. Teitelbaum, aren't you?" And I said, "Yes, and who the hell are you? Please put me down." And he said, "I had horrible back pain for decades. Nothing got rid of it, and I took your vitamin powder. It was gone in a month."

PEGGY: Wow!

DR TEITELBAUM: I designed the vitamin powder. My royalties all go to charity. I won't take money from any of the supplement companies.

PEGGY: Well, you know, just stop there for a minute. The concept of back pain being relieved by a powder... again, not an association that one would make. You wouldn't think, "I'm going to take a vitamin supplement to help my back pain."

DR TEITELBAUM: One day we'll need to do an interview on pain.

PEGGY: I'd like to.

DR TEITELBAUM: One out of three Americans suffer needlessly with chronic pain. Medications like Advil are found to kill 30,000 to 50,000 Americans needlessly each year, and herbals have been shown to be more effective than these medications in head-to-head studies. I like one called "Curamin," as a pain relief miracle, given six weeks to work. I'll use topical Comfry.

But here's the thing: Most pain is muscle pain. When muscles don't have enough energy, they're like a spring; they get stuck in the shortened position. You would think it's counterproductive. It takes energy to contract – but no. They contract when they need energy.

If you had a hard day of working out in the garden or whatever, you'd come home... you don't say, "Honey, my muscles are all just limp" because you had a hard day. You say, "They're all tight." When muscles don't have energy, they're like a spring; locked in the shortened position. And when they don't have enough energy chronically, they hurt.

And the most common cause of back pain, regardless of what you see in the X-ray, will be tight muscles. You give the muscles energy – the pain often goes away as the muscles release.

PEGGY: Could you just one more time tell us what was the miracle one? The –

DR TEITELBAUM: Curamin.

PEGGY: Curamin? And you take that for pain.

DR TEITELBAUM: Yes. Not Curcumin, but Curamin.

PEGGY: Curamin.

DR TEITELBAUM: That specific one. One to two, three times a day. You can take it with any pain medications. Give it six weeks. In the head-on studies with Celebrex, the people got more pain relief than they did with the Celebrex after the six weeks.

PEGGY: And I'm just going back to the start of this whole conversation about the importance of sleep. If you've dealt with pain, if back pain is keeping you up, or other pain is keeping you up at night, if you're taking this Curamin and your pain is being relieved, you may get into a deeper sleep. So you're on a good cycle there.

DR TEITELBAUM: And, if you sleep the pain will go away, because you make growth hormone, which basically is a repair system for muscles.

PEGGY: So all these things we're doing are feeding upon each other in a good, positive, constructive way.

DR TEITELBAUM: Synergy.

PEGGY: Right.

DR TEITELBAUM: Nutritional support – those simple things. And decrease excess sugar, except for chocolate. Chocolate's helpful…

PEGGY: I like that chocolate.

DR TEITELBAUM: And then "E" for exercise. Your body has a "use it or lose it" approach to efficiency. If you're not using it, your body's going to put it on hold. So go for walks, preferably in the sunshine. You don't have to dip yourself in sunscreen. The proper advice is to avoid sunburn, not sunshine. Your body needs the sunshine for the vitamin D.

PEGGY: For the vitamin D.

DR TEITELBAUM: Which is critical for many, many, many, many different things in the body. So if you optimize SHINE… and again, you can do the free energy analysis program at the www.endfatigue.com, which will take you through this – you will find that you're feeling dramatically better within three months.

PEGGY: So somebody who is feeling forgetful, feeling not as sharp, feeling senior moments, brain fog, all that – there's something they can do. None of this is terribly complicated.

DR TEITELBAUM: No, and you'll find that as you increase energy production in your brain, your brain is back.

PEGGY: Your brain is back. You're fast. You're processing. You're remembering. You're thinking. Your judgement is better –

DR TEITELBAUM: And your mood. You'll be happier.

PEGGY: Your mood. That is very important, and depression is, in fact, correlated with Alzheimer's.

DR TEITELBAUM: Yes, and let me mention two interesting studies on depression. They used a special form of curcumin, the same one that's in Curamin, although it's a different mix. The form is called "Curamed," and they gave 500 mg twice a day in people with depression, and they compared it to the antidepressant medication.

PEGGY: The prescription drugs.

DR TEITELBAUM: And the herbal Curamin, after six weeks, was more effective at relieving depression, especially severe depression, than the medication.

PEGGY: Very, very good to know. So we have many ways, none of them all that daunting, some of them very inexpensive.

DR TEITELBAUM: Most inexpensive.

PEGGY: And that we can use to tune up our brains. But the overall advice is, do find a doctor who's in sympathy with this approach, who's going to work with you.

DR TEITELBAUM: A holistic doctor.

PEGGY: Find a holistic doctor.

DR TEITELBAUM: Now, I do treat people from all over the world, most often by telephone, as long as they have their family doctor working with them to do an examination. But again, I'm not cheap. I'm a great value, but I'm pricey.

So for people with fibromyalgia and chronic fatigue syndrome and chronic pain, that's where I specialize. But for just a tune-up, go to www.aihm.org – not dot-com; dot-org. Or for a naturopathic physician, www.naturopathic.org.

PEGGY: And you can find somebody in your region...

DR TEITELBAUM: Over 4,000 people all over the country who know what they're doing here.

PEGGY: Who know what they're doing.

DR TEITELBAUM: As opposed to your family doctor who, nice person as they are, has no clue.

PEGGY: Has no clue. Well, Doctor, I want to thank you for coming because you have taken us through the SHINE Protocol and given us a whole new understanding of ways that we can energize our brain and clear away that brain fog, and be sharp and focused and optimistic and upbeat again, so I thank you so much.

DR TEITELBAUM: It's a pleasure, and again, 80 is the new 50.

PEGGY: 80's the new 50.

DR TEITELBAUM: Getting old is optional.

PEGGY: Getting old is optional. How great is that? Thank you so much for watching, and I hope you learned a lot – and you can learn more through Dr. Teitelbaum's smart phone app, "Cures A-Z," and his website, www.endfatigue.com. Thank you so much.

DR TEITELBAUM: I like the high-tech stuff!

PEGGY: Great, thank you.

Interview with Dr. David Perlmutter

PEGGY SARLIN: Hello, I'm Peggy Sarlin, and today I'm in Los Angeles, California, where I have the great pleasure of speaking with Dr. David Perlmutter, the renowned author of *Grain Brain* and *The Grain Brain Whole Life Plan*.

Dr. Perlmutter has really revolutionized our understanding of brain health. His books have been translated into 27 languages.

He is a board-certified neurologist and a fellow of the American College of Nutrition. So – neurology, nutrition... not a typical combination. He's the winner of the Linus Pauling Award for Neurological Innovations, and he's really a leader in educating the public about brain health. So welcome, Dr. Perlmutter.

DR. DAVID PERLMUTTER: Glad to be here. Thank you.

PEGGY: So Doctor, you're here in Los Angeles chairing the conference of the Institute for Functional Medicine on the dynamic brain. You're here with all these top brain experts. What are you hearing that's exciting and new, that's going to make us optimistic about our brain health?

DR PERLMUTTER: Well, I would say, first, it's not going to get us optimistic. It's going to reinforce the fact that we are, indeed, quite optimistic now.

The notion that the brain can grow new brain cells, for example, is brand new. That was only published in 1998. Before that, there had been this huge rejection of the notion that humans had a second chance.

And only in the past few years have we understood not just that we have this opportunity to grow new brain cells, but that, in addition, we can enhance the process.

These are brand-new cells. They are stem cells in the brain. So in a sense, we are seeing that stem cell therapy is happening in you and me, as we have this conversation. It happens when we are 80 years old, when we are 90 years old... It happens throughout our lifetimes.

It's a very empowering notion, because not only is it happening, but we can enhance the process through some very simple lifestyle changes.

PEGGY: So the whole notion of the brain as this kind of rusty engine that just deteriorates has been put by the wayside, and now this really is the paradigm shift. The brain is growing. It's new. It's continually in a state of rebirth. And people like you are figuring out that we know it can be reborn, new cells can grow – people like you are at the forefront of figuring how to do it – how to get us to do it in a practical way.

DR PERLMUTTER: That's right, and this is research going on worldwide, in which people are looking at questions like how do you amplify the growth of new brain cells, and, in addition, support the differentiation of those brain cells so they become specialized?

And even further, how do you amplify this process we call "neuroplasticity" that allows one cell to connect to another and redirect its growth, etc.?

We know one chemical that happens to be really fundamental mechanistically in making this happen, allowing it to happen, is called "BDNF." Now, that sounds a bit technical, but go with me on this.

PEGGY: Oh, I'm with you. Take me away on BDNF.

DR PERLMUTTER: BDNF is basically growth hormone for the brain. And when you have higher levels of BDNF, as research has demonstrated, you are resistant to getting Alzheimer's in the first place.

When it comes to your rate of cognitive decline over many years – with the image that you mentioned earlier of a rusting brain really being something we will put by the wayside – we now know higher levels of BDNF correlate with slower decline of the brain.

In fact, newer research correlates actual growth of the brain's memory center over one to two years in people with the highest level of BDNF, and that is revolutionary. You know, we all sort of accepted the notion that as we age, our brains will rust, as you mentioned, deteriorate, and shrink, and lose the ability to function.

We now understand this just isn't true. And it's taken a lot for people to embrace this as it relates to the brain, because we still tend to cling to this notion that we peak out around 18 years of age, and then after that it's "We're all on the skids." You know, you drink a beer, and that's 30,000 brain cells, and the next thing you know, you're in deep trouble when you're 50, or 60, or 80.

PEGGY: That's so depressing.

DR PERLMUTTER: But that just isn't what our science is telling us anymore; what it's telling us is that when we amplify this chemical, BDNF, then we get a second chance. We suddenly turn things around, and the brain regenerates itself. And that is clearly a revolutionary concept.

PEGGY: So let's stay with BDNF. Can we consider it almost a youth hormone?

DR PERLMUTTER: Well, as it relates to the brain, you've got it. That's for sure.

PEGGY: So if BDNF is this magical elixir that's going to grow our brain cells for us – new brain cells – how do we be good to our brains? What are these lifestyle interventions that are going to encourage the production of it?

DR PERLMUTTER: It's a great question, because one thing that people are able to do to have higher levels of BDNF is very, very expensive. They have to go out and buy a pair of sneakers. And once they do, and not just buy the sneakers, but use them...

PEGGY: Oh!

DR PERLMUTTER: In other words, aerobic exercise.

PEGGY: Specifically, aerobic.

DR PERLMUTTER: The most powerful way to change your DNA, so that your DNA begins to express this protein, this brain-derived neurotrophic factor BDNF, is exercise.

Much of the research was done in Pittsburgh, but much was actually done right here in Los Angeles, where you and I are, at UCLA, demonstrating dramatic changes in memory, increasing the volume of the brain's memory center, and all correlated with higher levels of BDNF in comparisons between those individuals who exercise versus those who do not.

So while everybody already knows that exercise makes you feel good...

PEGGY: Makes you look better.

DR PERLMUTTER: Makes you look better; you develop endorphins, so you enjoy life; maybe it's better for your bone density, if you're a woman...

But now we correlate your degree of participation in aerobic exercise with the growth of new brain cells, the increase in size of your brain's memory center, and better cognitive function. All you gotta do is exercise. You know, there is such a push for...

PEGGY: Wow!

DR PERLMUTTER: ...this or that new proprietary drug, or "this is in development," or connecting your brain to a computer, and trying to upload information, and all these new technologies...

The bottom line is, get out and huff and puff a little bit, and you're going to dramatically improve structurally what the brain looks like, and functionally what your brain is able to do.

PEGGY: Well, you're specifying aerobic. So obviously, there are other kinds of exercise, and they may have merits – lifting weights, stretching...but you're saying aerobic.

DR PERLMUTTER: It turns out that resistance exercise is effective as well. And ultimately, what the main researchers, led by a guy named Dr. Kirk Erickson, have revealed is that it's basically your caloric expenditure in doing whatever you like.

It can be dancing. It can be walking, swimming, biking, jogging...you name it, but as long as you're burning calories, the more calories you burn, the better.

So what an incredible thought it is that people get a second chance; that you can go out and have stem cell therapy today, just by exercising.

PEGGY: Wow! Well, for people like me that's exciting...because frankly, I don't like to exercise. So you're telling me I can keep my brain young and get this gorgeous BDNF flowing inside my brain structures, and that's motivating me.

But I just want to do the bare minimum. And there's got to be other people like me out there. So tell me the minimum.

DR PERLMUTTER: Well, there are other people like you who may not wish to participate in aerobics, I would accept your statement, but I would do everything I could to convince you that you need to exercise. Why? Because as you sit here right now, you are at risk for Alzheimer's. If you live to be age 85, your risk is 50-50.

PEGGY: 50-50.

DR PERLMUTTER: You are a woman. That means your risk is much greater than mine. And certainly, if there's a family history, indeed, your risk is even higher.

We have no treatment. There's no pharmaceutical treatment that works for that disease that currently affects 5.4 million Americans. And it's costing us more than $230 billion a year.

Having said that, I'm not going to accept your complaint that you don't like to exercise. However, I know where you're going with this, and I think it's to a place of, "Well, in addition, Doctor, what else is there that scientific research has demonstrated will also raise BDNF?" And there are actually a number of things.

There are various herbs that have an effect on BDNF – like turmeric, for example. Turmeric, the Indian spice, up-regulates BDNF, increases BDNF. The Omega-3 fatty acid called DHA works quite handily, which is why fish is considered brain food.

There are new things that have been researched that are going to be available soon. For example, whole coffee fruit concentrate. What is that? When you buy your coffee beans, you're actually getting the seed of the coffee berry. But the rest of that coffee berry, the pulp of that fruit, has now been studied and known to be a powerful source of BDNF.

Being on a diet that is more what we call "keto.".. In other words, burning more fat than carbs, generally, increases the body's BDNF by its production of a chemical called "beta hydroxy butyrate." And also, butyrate in general – a fat, if you will, a ketone – increases BDNF. Where do we get that? We get butyrate in our bodies from our gut bacteria fermenting fiber-rich foods that we may eat.

So what did I just say?

PEGGY: A lot.

DR PERLMUTTER: I just connected the gut bacteria to growing new brain cells, what we call the gut-brain connection – that a healthy array of gut bacteria, when they are fed appropriately with what we call "prebiotic fiber" (we'll talk about those foods in just a moment) produce a chemical called "butyrate" that actually speeds up the body's production of BDNF, and helps you grow new brain cells.

That is our powerful relationship between our cognitive future and the health of the bugs that live in the gut.

PEGGY: Which is a totally mind-blowing idea that you have really brought to public attention, I think you have more than anybody else,

So just going back to our theme here of consciously trying to structure our lives so we're promoting the BDNF production in our brain. We know we're going to exercise, even if we don't want to. We're going to buy the sneakers. And we have to do that every day, seven days a week? How often?

DR PERLMUTTER: I would love seven days a week. Well, sometimes we travel, and for whatever reason, it's not possible. But personally I have found it's always easy to make an excuse, you know?

PEGGY: Yeah, it is.

DR PERLMUTTER: But the truth of the matter is, there's probably not a hotel that you might be in any more that doesn't have some type of gym equipment. You can bring a pair of walking shoes with you, get out wherever you go and take a walk – and *always* find time to get out. So I'm not going to let you off the hook. There are no excuses. I mean, if it's six days a week, that's fine.

PEGGY: But is it 15 minutes a day? Is it a half hour...?

DR PERLMUTTER: I think 20 minutes is reasonable.

PEGGY: 20 minutes.

DR PERLMUTTER: New research is actually indicating closer to 45 minutes to an hour. That is an investment in the future of your brain. And if we're talking about reversing Alzheimer's, that's certainly one powerful component to the program.

But if an individual has already been diagnosed with Alzheimer's, the truth of the matter is that there is limited scope to provide anything that is going to have a dramatic effect in terms of reversing it. Although now we're seeing that when we leverage multiple ideas – bringing in nutrition issues, hormone balancing, detoxification, aerobic exercise, the stabilization of certain blood parameters like homocysteine, vitamin D levels, for example...in short, when multiple issues are considered, we do see that now it's possible, in many patients, to reverse Alzheimer's disease.

And that is a heck of a statement that a few years ago I wouldn't have been able to make, but it's now happening, and it's very exciting.

PEGGY: Now you can make it.

DR PERLMUTTER: My mission, however, is to certainly fan the flames of that mentality. But beyond that, I believe what is much more important is to spread the word that we now understand that Alzheimer's is a preventable disease in the first place. While it's great that we target Alzheimer's in terms of therapeutic approaches...

PEGGY: Right.

DR PERLMUTTER: ...if we can keep it from happening in the first place, that makes a heck of a lot more sense. Because once the house is on fire, people will come and try to put the fire out, but why don't we go through the house, first of all, and make sure we didn't leave the iron on, and that the fireplace doesn't have some burning embers? And then we're able to walk away peacefully.

We can prevent Alzheimer's, by and large. Individuals, for example, who engage in aerobic exercise may have as much as a 50% reduction for that very disease for which there is no pharmaceutical fix. Individuals who do not develop Type II diabetes may have as much as a 50% reduction in the risk for Alzheimer's.

A new study published in the journal *JAMA Neurology* showed that those people who chronically take acid-blocking drugs called "proton pump inhibitors" that everybody thinks they need to take, have a 44% increased risk for developing Alzheimer's-type dementia.

PEGGY: That's very scary.

DR PERLMUTTER: It's scary. It's information that needs to get out. And again, it's not that you're just interviewing Dr. Perlmutter today, and he comes up with these ideas. That was published in the journal *JAMA Neurology,* put out by the American Medical Association. We need to talk about that stuff.

PEGGY: And if you go to your doctor, and he gives you this medication, is he going to say to you, "By the way, this is dramatically increasing your risk of Alzheimer's"? I mean, does it come with a warning?

DR PERLMUTTER: I think it's extremely unlikely. I lectured yesterday to a very large audience of healthcare providers, and when I put up that data, nobody in the audience seemed to have ever seen it.

PEGGY: Really?

DR PERLMUTTER: So it is our mission to get that information out. It's published data. An extremely large study showing not only an increased risk for Alzheimer's, but also a dramatically increased risk for other issues. Another study, a Stanford study, demonstrated a 16% increased risk for heart attack, and doubling of the risk of death from that event. So...

PEGGY: How dreadful!

DR PERLMUTTER: Yes. So we really need to do our best. You know, the word "doctor" doesn't mean healer. It means teacher. So the mission, by and large, is getting out there in venues like this, and letting people know the other side of the story that you're not going to see on the commercial when you watch the evening news.

In the case of these proton pump inhibitors, in the commercials it's all about acid indigestion, or you can't eat a certain food? Take this pill, and the world is gonna be a better place.

PEGGY: Right.

DR PERLMUTTER: That's not reality.

PEGGY: That's not reality.

DR PERLMUTTER: Reality is, you've increased your risk for Alzheimer's by about 44%.

PEGGY: I'm just kind of curious. I don't know if you know the answer to this, but I keep coming back to BDNF, because it seems to be so central to everything. Would these medications affect the production or discourage the production of BDNF? Is that the mechanism?

DR PERLMUTTER: That's a terrific question. And what we know is that there is this balance going on in the body between, on the one hand, the growth of new brain cells stimulated by BDNF, and then, on the other hand, a mechanism called "inflammation." So that's the balance.

When we do things that increase inflammation, we compromise the brain's vitality, the brain's ability to rejuvenate itself. On the other hand, when we are exercising, taking turmeric, taking DHA, or whole coffee fruit concentrate, then we are enhancing the brain's ability to rejuvenate itself, and to resist decline, i.e., reduce our risk for Alzheimer's and other neurodegenerative conditions.

PEGGY: It's interesting that you said a few years ago you couldn't have made the statement that it's now possible to actually reverse Alzheimer's. But now it is because of this programmatic way that you're looking at it. It's not the magic pill. It's a case of, you can address this issue, this imbalance, this problem here.

And that's what you've been laying out with us, in parallel with the production BDNF – a series of programs.

So just to keep reviewing, we're going to exercise, and then we're going to take supplements. I mean, that is a good idea, right? The whole subject of supplements is so confusing, because every doctor has their own particular favorites, and it can get expensive and confusing to people.

So if you were putting together something like the equivalent of a basic wardrobe – the jeans, the Navy blazer – what's like your basic wardrobe, of BDNF...?

DR PERLMUTTER: Well, the first very, very important supplement, probably on the top of the list of all the supplements you would add, would be one called "exercise."

PEGGY: I'm glad you're emphasizing that!

DR PERLMUTTER: And I'm not going to let it go. I'm just not going to let it go.

PEGGY: No, no, no. You're motivating me. You're motivating me.

DR PERLMUTTER: Because it is hugely powerful from a mechanistic perspective. We see the research that shows increasing size of the brain's memory center, and improved memory, with just one intervention, and that is the aerobic exercise.

PEGGY: Are we talking about the hippocampus?

DR PERLMUTTER: Yes, growth of the hippocampus in those who exercise, and resistance to Alzheimer's. I mean, what more could a person want to hear in a venue like this?

But beyond that, I believe that we've gotta maximize our understanding of the importance, for example, of vitamin D.

People will go to the doctor, and he or she will check blood level for vitamin D, and people will walk out being told they are "in the normal range." That is not meaningful, or really, very appropriate anymore, because "in the normal range" doesn't really tell you that you've optimized your situation, but you might just be scraping by.

If the normal range is between 30 and 90, or 30 to 100, depending on the lab, and you have a 32, your doctor may say, "Well, you're in the normal range. Go home. Everything's fine."

That's not what's best for you. You're scraping by. We like vitamin D levels up towards the top end, up around 80 or 90.

We want to make sure that your blood test for homocysteine, for example, is low. We don't like homocysteine levels that are high, because well-performed scientific research has correlated elevated levels of this amino acid, if you will, homocysteine, with higher risk for Alzheimer's and shrinkage of the brain's memory center.

We want to make sure that your average blood sugar is lower, as measured by the A1C. Many people are familiar with that. Well-published research has demonstrated that the higher the A1C, the greater is the decline in size of your hippocampus. So we want to make sure your A1C is lower, indicating that your average blood sugar is lower. Fasting insulin should be low.

These are all important parameters that are really straightforward. There is nothing exotic about these that would mean a doctor wouldn't be able to check them.

Certainly, there are other more exotic and perhaps a little bit more challenging laboratory studies, like looking at toxicology, looking at hormone levels, etc., that I think are very important as well, but might not be an area of familiarity for most typical doctors or even neurologists who may be seeing patients at risk for cognitive decline, or seeing those patients who already have mild cognitive impairment.

They are nonetheless very, very important. They're not typically on the menu at the standard neurological evaluation.

PEGGY: Right.

DR PERLMUTTER: But we're hoping to change that. We're hoping to spread the recognition that these parameters can have important roles to play in determining the destiny of a person's brain.

And not only are they interesting to look at, but much more importantly, they can be fixed. They provide actionable information, information about what you can do.

If the vitamin D is low, here's how you fix it, then recheck it. If the homocysteine is high, you take the B-6, B-12, and folic acid, and repeat your study to make sure homocytsteine is normalized. If the C-reactive protein is elevated, let's engage dietary changes, etc., to reduce inflammation, and follow the C-reactive protein as a marker of that inflammation.

We will look at lipopolysaccharide, LPS, as a marker of leakiness of the gut, and inflammation – again, tying gut health to brain health, which for me as a neurologist is certainly nothing that was in the playbook just a few years ago.

The point is, there is no silver bullet here.

PEGGY: Right.

DR PERLMUTTER: As Dr. Bredesen likes to talk about, it's "silver buckshot," meaning there are multiple areas that need to be paid attention to in order to bring about change.

The brain doesn't decline just because one thing is askew. Multiple things conspire to create an environment in which the brain then is unable to thrive. That said, you have to target as many of those entities as possible, if you're going to reverse Alzheimer's disease.

PEGGY: Speaking of the real world and the situations people actually run into as they try to implement this, older people are the people who are more at risk of cognition problems, and so exercise would be great for them.

But they might have physical problems. They might have back problems. They might have knee problems. How are you going to help them get the exercise they need? Give us advice for those people.

DR PERLMUTTER: It's a terrific question, and I would say that there are some excuses just now that have been put forth, and I'm not buying it. I mean, I'm in the gym next to people who have terrible knee issues, with multiple knee operations, and they're on a machine that allows them to become aerobic, based on using their upper extremities. You know, it's like a bicycle for the arms.

PEGGY: Right.

DR PERLMUTTER: There are so many things that people are able to do. Some people are terribly out of shape, and unable to tolerate going out and jogging three miles. I understand that.

PEGGY: Right.

DR PERLMUTTER: But you could jog two miles, or one mile... or walk one block... or walk from your front door to the mailbox, as a start... or walk from the bedroom back into the living room a couple of times, to start.

There's always a way to do more than you're doing right now. Be aware of the notion that being so sedentary for eleven hours a day is leading to a brain that's just not going to be functional, and more importantly, it's going to be at much more risk for decline. And you know, that's why we're here.

PEGGY: That's why we're here. Okay, we know in our program we've got exercise. We've got supplements. And we know we're going to eat great – and that involves the care and feeding of our gut bacteria.

DR PERLMUTTER: Exactly. That was a very powerful statement just now. We're going to eat right, and it involves the care and feeding of our gut bacteria. It is really a new perspective.

I wrote a book called *Brain Maker* that really deals with the important role of gut bacteria in brain health. Who knew? Well, who knows are the scientists from around the world who have now recognized this critical role of our gut bacteria in determining the health of the human brain.

It's a very humbling but yet empowering bit of science to embrace, because it opens the door to our ability to leverage this science and create programs that will enhance brain health.

Our gut bacteria really determine the set point of inflammation in the human body. When we recognize that inflammation is a primary feature of brain degeneration in Alzheimer's... in Parkinson's... in Huntington's... in multiple sclerosis... in autism...

PEGGY: Autism.

DR PERLMUTTER: Targeting inflammation at its source is really something that becomes of fundamental importance. Again, inflammation has its genesis as a consequence of changes in the gut bacteria. This leads to increased permeability of the gut lining, and that allows a variety of things, including bacteria themselves, to get through the gut lining and challenge the immune system, creating the chemical mediators of inflammation that do get into the brain and begin this process that leads to brain cells virtually committing suicide – a process called "apoptosis" in which these cells basically just die, and we suffer decline as a consequence of that.

On the other side of that scale is the growth of new brain cells, which is enhanced by anything that will enhance BDNF, as we talked about.

PEGGY: So what we eat determines the health of our brain. I mean, it's just so basic.

DR PERLMUTTER: It is, and it's kind of cute to talk about that, but I can assure you that that notion is founded and supported by our most well-respected scientific institutions, publishing in the most well-respected peer-reviewed journals.

As an example, in a recent publication in the *Journal of Alzheimer's Disease* (what a name for a journal!), researchers from the Mayo Clinic looked at the diets of individuals, and essentially asked, "What do these people eat, and what was their risk of developing dementia?"

What they found was really quite interesting: that those individuals who favored carbohydrates as their highest source of calorie input had about an 80 to 85% increased risk of developing dementia. Those individuals whose diets favored more fat as a caloric resource had about a 44% risk reduction, in terms of Alzheimer's dementia.

So that tells you that this idea of castigation of fat as a dietary input, which has really quite characterized the American recommendations, and spread across the globe, was really off base, at least as it relates to the brain, and now we know better, really, as relates to the health of the human body, including heart health.

We've eaten fat as a powerful source of calories for a couple of million years. Suddenly, 30 years ago, fat was demonized.

PEGGY: The villain!

DR PERLMUTTER: That's right.

PEGGY: The ultimate villain.

DR PERLMUTTER: We're told eat low-fat, no fat this and that...

PEGGY: Right.

DR PERLMUTTER: Which by default, caused people to eat more carbs. Rates of heart disease and diabetes and cancer and Alzheimer's have gone up dramatically since that has been the dogma.

PEGGY: Right.

DR PERLMUTTER: And now, gratefully, even the United States' dietary recommendations have changed, indicating that the biggest problem in our diet has really been the sugar and the carbs all along, and not the fat.

Which is not to say that certain fats are not dangerous. Certainly, they are. The vegetable fats, the corn oils and safflower oils that line the grocery store shelves are really to be avoided, because they're not good for us. They do increase inflammation.

But fish oil, the oils that are found in nuts and seeds, grass-fed beef and wild fish, for example, are terrific for us, because they actually can help us reduce inflammation. And many of those oils do, in fact, increase BDNF. Why wouldn't we want to have those on board?

The other really critically important part of the puzzle relates back to something we mentioned earlier, and that is nurturing the gut bacteria. We nurture our gut bacteria and reduce inflammation and cater to the brain by having higher levels in our diets of what is called "prebiotic fiber."

PEGGY: And most of us don't know that. This is a new concept to many people.

DR PERLMUTTER: Well, everyone's heard that fiber-rich foods are good for us, because they're good for digestion and who knows what else?

PEGGY: But the prebiotic fiber idea is new to me.

DR PERLMUTTER: Exactly. "Prebiotic" sort of sounds like probiotic.

PEGGY: Right.

DR PERLMUTTER: And it's good that they sound similar. Why? Because they're very much in the same camp. Probiotics are the good bacteria, and prebiotics are what they eat.

We get prebiotic fiber from eating prebiotic fiber-rich foods like Mexican yam, which is jicama, garlic, onions, leeks, dandelion greens, asparagus... Those are foods rich in prebiotic fiber. Chicory root.

But more importantly, as part of the nutritional supplement program, you can go to your favorite health food store and stand there and say, "I want some prebiotic fiber," and they'll likely provide you a product that's made from acacia gum.

Acacia is the big canopy tree in Africa, where you see the giraffe in the noon-day sun seeking shelter. And that tree secretes a gum, a resin that is sustainably harvested, powdered, put in a bag, and ends up on the health food store shelf. You take a teaspoon twice a day of that prebiotic fiber, and you're nurturing your gut bacteria, allowing them to produce this chemical I mentioned earlier called butyrate, which is just manna for the brain.

PEGGY: So maybe in our basic wardrobe of supplements that we were talking about, which had turmeric, and the fish oil, and maybe vitamin D, maybe we should add to our basic list a prebiotic fiber.

DR PERLMUTTER: Oh, yup, sure. I wasn't done with that, that's for sure.

PEGGY: Oh, okay.

DR PERLMUTTER: So that's a great list that you're developing.

PEGGY: Yes, yes, okay.

DR PERLMUTTER: And let's just recap for a moment. It would be DHA, the Omega-3 found in fish and fish oils. There is even...

PEGGY: Or krill oils, or...

DR PERLMUTTER: Krill oil, even a vegetarian form that's on the market. That's really fundamental, even for children. I mean, the richest source of DHA in nature is human breast milk.

PEGGY: Oh, well that tells you something.

DR PERLMUTTER: That just gives you a sense of how important that is for the brain. Vitamin D I think is critically important.

PEGGY: How much, by the way?

DR PERLMUTTER: Well, again, that depends on the blood test. There's a little bit of manipulation, a little bit of integration that has to happen with you as an individual. You might be out in the sun day in and day out with no clothes on, running around your neighborhood, in which case, you may not need a vitamin D supplement.

PEGGY: Unlikely.

DR PERLMUTTER: On the other hand, you may live in the Northeast, or the Northwest, where you're not getting a lot of sun exposure in the winter, you're wearing a lot of clothing, and therefore, your body's not manufacturing vitamin D. You'll need more than somebody who lives in a sunnier climate...

PEGGY: So what would be the range? I mean, a range for somebody who's, let's say, in the Northeast, not outside, working a desk job... ?

DR PERLMUTTER: You know, again, people who begin taking vitamin D should have their levels followed by blood tests.

PEGGY: Okay.

DR PERLMUTTER: Taking 2,000 IU a day for you might be enough, but might not be enough for me. I might need 5,000, or even 10,000 units a day.

PEGGY: Wow, that's a lot.

DR PERLMUTTER: Who knows? It isn't a lot.

PEGGY: Oh, okay.

DR PERLMUTTER: It might be just right. 1,000 units is not a little. It might be just right. But the only way you're going to know is by blood testing.

PEGGY: Okay, so that's important.

DR PERLMUTTER: Similarly, we know that the B vitamins are really important, because they lower homocysteine. But, for example, if your homocysteine is very high, like 18, you would need more of those B vitamins, following the homocysteine level by tests until it normalizes. So that's where we apply a little bit of interventional science and medicine into this relationship.

PEGGY: Right. You're not just guessing scattershot...

DR PERLMUTTER: Right. It's personalized medicine.

PEGGY: It's personalized medicine.

DR PERLMUTTER: It's not what I need, but what do you need?

PEGGY: Yeah, that's the future.

DR PERLMUTTER: And how do I know what you need? Real simple. We have wonderful laboratory studies that'll tell me right now what you need. So vitamin D – important. Turmeric – been studied...

Actually, one of the prime researchers, Dr. Cole, is located right here in Los Angeles and has researched turmeric in its multiple activities. We know that turmeric increases BDNF. It helps to reduce the load of plaque in the brain, at least in laboratory animals. We know that people who have higher levels of turmeric in their diets, by virtue of the fact that they eat a lot of curried foods, have a lower risk for dementia as well.

These are all interesting sidelights that I think play into the notion that turmeric is really important for the brain. And that's brand-new information. It was only just published 2,000 years ago in the Vedic texts, that turmeric is good for your vitality, and also for your brain.

PEGGY: Only 2,000 years. Only 2,000 years.

DR PERLMUTTER: I think alpha lipoic acid is an important supplement.

PEGGY: ALA.

DR PERLMUTTER: NAC, N-acetyl cysteine, coenzyme Q10 – very important. I think there's clearly a role for a very high quality probiotic supplement, with multiple strains – you know, 10, 15 strains of bacteria, as well as a high-concentration – you know, 30 billion, 50 billion colony-forming units. That's what you want to look for on the label.

But the most important thing to look for on the label of a probiotic is its stability. Is it delivering to you those organisms after six months, after a year?

PEGGY: How do you know?

DR PERLMUTTER: Well, one thing you can look for is if they say, "Our product has 30 billion at the time of manufacture..."

PEGGY: 30 billion – these numbers are staggering. Okay.

DR PERLMUTTER: Well, they're not. These are microscopic organisms.

PEGGY: Right.

DR PERLMUTTER: So... It might say, "at the time of manufacture," but I want 30 billion units to be guaranteed for me as long as I have that product on the shelf, and I'm taking it.

PEGGY: Okay.

DR PERLMUTTER: So that's one thing you would look for.

I think non-GMO is also a plus. And not to underestimate the importance of prebiotic fiber, especially as we're talking about what you would add to your nutritional supplements.

That's a new player, a new kid on the block, because people haven't really heard about this. But to nurture your gut bacteria with prebiotic fiber – great. Eat those foods that I enumerated earlier. But in addition, we know that you really need to help that along, because you can't eat enough prebiotic fiber just by food. You're really going to have to eat an awful lot of Mexican yam, garlic, onions, leeks... Take the fiber.

Again, there are a lot of things. One of the most exciting is this whole coffee fruit concentrate.

PEGGY: Is it available on the market now?

DR PERLMUTTER: It will be available, yes.

PEGGY: It will be, or...?

DR PERLMUTTER: It will be very, very soon. The research is out now. In fact, at this conference I put some slides up and talked about how exciting that is. But we're seeing that that's going to be available in health food stores. It's called "whole coffee fruit concentrate," and indeed, along the lines of exercise, DHA, turmeric, it's yet another player in terms of increasing BDNF.

Now, there is one other supplement that is now getting a lot of attention and it is sage.

PEGGY: Yes, sage.

DR PERLMUTTER: Everybody grows sage. You see it. People have it in their gardens. There are a couple of forms. There's one called sage "officinalis," which is common sage. That's the Latin name. And there's a bucket of research now showing that that's good for the brain as well.

It actually has some activity that works along the lines to increase a certain brain transmitter called "acetylcholine." But like the other things I've mentioned, it, too, enhances BDNF.

We'll see more about sage in the future, but there are supplements of sage that you can go to your health food store and buy right now. Various brands offer it, and you could take that, and it's good for your brain.

PEGGY: That's very good to know. You didn't name that many supplements. We're not too intimidated.

Just going back to the whole idea of what we're supposed to eat on a daily basis – you've been so key to educating the public about the low carb, higher fat approach to eating. Is there a resistance you've run into? Are there misconceptions about the needs for carbohydrates, like, "Oh, you're hurting your body by depriving it of carbs"?

DR PERLMUTTER: We all grew up in a time when we were told, "You need to have a candy bar before you take your SATs." Why? Because the brain needs a lot of glucose. And it was one of the things that was sort of indelible, wasn't it, that dietary fat was bad?

PEGGY: Yes.

DR PERLMUTTER: Remember those days?

PEGGY: Yeah.

DR PERLMUTTER: And your brain needs glucose.

Well, as a matter of fact, the human brain functions far more efficiently, and ultimately better, when it is powering itself with fat, and not sugar.

So this notion of loading up with sugar because it's good for your brain is contrary to what our best research is telling us.

In the long run, when you're eating sugar, and your blood sugar ultimately continues to rise, that is hugely threatening for your brain. In a study that appeared in *The New England Journal* in September of 2013, they took a group of about 3,000 individuals and simply checked their blood sugar at the beginning of the study. They followed them for several years. Then they went back, and they determined who developed dementia and who did not.

What they found was that those who developed dementia had higher blood sugar at the beginning of the study. And what was really compelling was the fact that their blood sugars weren't really anything that most doctors would worry about – 100 to 105. 105 blood sugar was already associated with increased risk for dementia.

Blood sugar elevation happens when we eat sugar, so we've got to stop eating this white powder that is more addictive than other white powders that people were so fearful of, in terms of addiction, throughout the years. This is the most worrisome white powder on the planet – sugar.

The people really need to be aware of hidden sources of sugar, like a glass of orange juice. You know, your 12-ounce glass of OJ has nine teaspoons of sugar. Those 36 grams of carbs are really detrimental, especially if you're trying to limit your carbs to 60 to 80 a day.

Two glasses of orange juice in the morning and you've already hit your level of carbs for the entire day. Not to say that all carbs are bad. Complex carbohydrate, like the type we get in prebiotic fiber, is, of course, really good for the brain.

So what do people do when they hear this messaging about avoiding sugar? "I shouldn't be drinking sugar-sweetened sodas, so what would be a good choice? Diet drinks." Well, does that make sense?

Just six weeks ago, a study was published showing that those individuals who drink one or more diet drinks a day – artificially sweetened, no sugar, no calories – almost triple their risk for developing Alzheimer's disease.

PEGGY: Ah! That's so scary.

DR PERLMUTTER: They have at least doubled their risk for diabetes, and have a huge increased risk for becoming obese, by drinking a beverage with no sugar, and no calories. The reason is because of the dramatic changes in the gut bacteria that occur from artificial sweetener consumption. It all comes back to roost, doesn't it?

PEGGY: Is there any beverage that we can think that will promote BDNF?

DR PERLMUTTER: That will promote BDNF... well, a great beverage to drink is water. Fruit-flavored water, I think, is terrific. There are drinks you see in the health food store that have lots of turmeric in them. Ashwagandha...

PEGGY: Oh, there you go.

DR PERLMUTTER: Drinking kombucha, for example, helps the gut bacteria. It's a bit of a probiotic type of drink. And as I've mentioned now, the gut bacteria play a role in creating this chemical called butyrate, which enhances BDNF production. So, sure, drink kombucha. I prefer to water it down.

Tea, coffee...coffee is a wonderful way in the morning of increasing your body's production of beta hydroxy butyrate, another form of butyrate. It's the reason that the ketogenic diet, getting the body into a state of ketosis, has become so popular, because people are seeing really dramatic changes in their health when they finally get off the sugar and carbs and eat more fat.

PEGGY: The last time we spoke, you told me that you start your day with just coffee, your coffee, and I think you put coconut oil in it.

DR PERLMUTTER: I do.

PEGGY: And now I do that.

DR PERLMUTTER: I often do.

PEGGY: That's my breakfast.

DR PERLMUTTER: Well, there you go. You know, a study was published six weeks ago on the role of caffeine consumption, in terms of increasing the production of this butyrate, beta hydroxy butyrate.

Having said that, I don't want people to get the wrong message – while a cup of coffee is good, that doesn't necessarily mean that these creative drinks that you'll get at the coffee shop, with the whipped cream, and the...

PEGGY: Oh, well, sugar.

DR PERLMUTTER: Yes, and all these things are going to be good for you.

PEGGY: Artificial flavors, all that stuff.

DR PERLMUTTER: That's not your cup of coffee. There's one that's offered at a very popular coffee global store, something "ino," or "cino.".. I don't know what it is. I'm not going to say what it is, but nonetheless it has 70 grams of sugar and 76 grams of carbs in one. So that will not help you get into ketosis, and it's not really healthy.

PEGGY: That is not brain-friendly food.

DR PERLMUTTER: Well said.

PEGGY: With your emphasis on fats, you're taking us into the area of ketones and the ketogenic diet, and is that something you recommend?

DR PERLMUTTER: I think that spending some time in ketosis on a daily basis is something most people do anyway. Generally, you wake up in a mild state of ketosis. Let's see if we can protract that, and that is to say, by not having breakfast, for example.

Wow! You know, I am certainly sounding iconoclastic by saying that we shouldn't eat breakfast. Didn't Mom tell you that that's the most important meal of the day, and loaded us up with carbs so that we could go to school and do well? You know, the short stack of pancakes with the maple syrup, which was probably never maple syrup in the first place.

PEGGY: That was Mom love!

DR PERLMUTTER: But that said, the longer we can extend the nighttime fast, I think, is good. Have breakfast a couple days a week. Have it five days a week, but take a couple of days each week and don't have breakfast. Have your first meal at noon or two o'clock. Your body will thank you for that, and you'll reestablish a connection with what it feels like to be hungry.

Few people these days really ever experience hunger anymore. It's good to reestablish a signaling mechanism in your body that tells you it's time to eat, as opposed to breakfast, lunch and dinner, three meals a day. Somebody invented that three meals routine. That didn't just happen.

PEGGY: I like that!

DR PERLMUTTER: Because there have been efforts on both sides of the story, saying, "Well, we shouldn't have three meals a day. We should have six meals a day."

PEGGY: Break it down into little ones, yeah.

DR PERLMUTTER: Right, so that our blood sugar doesn't spike and our insulin levels don't spike, and it'll cause you to have less risk for insulin resistance.

Others like myself are saying, "Miss a meal here and there. Fast for an entire day – good for you." It's a low level of stress on your body that we call "hormesis" that's actually good for you. It allows certain life-sustaining genes to express themselves, and code for chemicals that are antioxidant, that are detoxicant, that are increasing your ability to deal with inflammation.

This is a good thing to do, and it emulates what the diets of our ancestors must have been like.

PEGGY: They didn't have refrigerators.

DR PERLMUTTER: You know, hunting and gathering doesn't mean hunting down a convenience store, and gathering up all of the chips.

There are times when our hunter-gatherer forbears didn't have a meal. They weren't going to stop chasing the gazelle to hunt it down because "It's lunchtime, and we're on break." It didn't happen that way. You went until you finally were able to achieve food.

PEGGY: And that's what our bodies are designed to do.

DR PERLMUTTER: That's right. Well, it's what our genes expect.

Our lifestyle and particularly our foods influence, from moment to moment, our gene expression. So by missing a meal, we change the expression of our genome to allow the expression of genes that help code for longevity and brain preservation.

PEGGY: You know, I want to go back to something you said. You used the word "stress." You said if we do this kind of extended fast, we're lessening the stress on our body. In your book – I should say, your very fine book, *The Grain Brain Whole Life Plan* – you talk about stress, stress in the brain, and the necessity of getting a handle on stress so that it doesn't corrode the brain, essentially. So can you help us understand that?

DR PERLMUTTER: Delighted to. You know, it's a stressful world in which we live.

PEGGY: Yes.

DR PERLMUTTER: And when we are under stress, it is really dysfunctional for the brain.

If you want to be mechanistic about it, we know that higher levels of stress are associated with higher levels of a chemical called "cortisol." What does cortisol do? Cortisol increases the leakiness of the gut, which amplifies inflammation. It changes the array of organisms in the gut, it changes for the worse the bacterial diversity that we have.

And higher levels of cortisol are directly toxic to the brain's memory center, as was wonderfully described by Dr. Robert Sapolsky, also out here in California.

PEGGY: Oh, this is the place to be.

DR PERLMUTTER: This is the place to be.

PEGGY: This is the brain place.

DR PERLMUTTER: So what can you do? You can turn off the TV. You can reduce your engagement with all of the stressful news that is everywhere we turn.

PEGGY: Yes, it's hard to turn it off. We're being bombarded with it.

DR PERLMUTTER: Sure. I mean, you go to a hotel. You're going to take the elevator downstairs to go to a conference, and – as if you might miss something – in the elevator is a television on with the news about how terrible the world is.

PEGGY: None of the news is good. Yeah.

DR PERLMUTTER: So offload stress by engaging in meditation, by engaging in exercise, and by disengaging from the bombardment we get day in and day out by the threats that are clearly out there, that we just don't need to engage.

The other thing that's really vitally important, as it relates to brain health, is getting restorative sleep. It's so highly underrated, the notion that sleep makes you feel good – great. But sleep is a brain tonic, and it's really important to recognize that the quality of our sleep matters in ways that are almost indescribable.

People may think they're sleeping well, but in reality the five hours that they're getting a night is not enough. Or they may think they're sleeping for eight hours, but in reality, that sleep is very interruptive, and not restorative.

The only way you're going to know is by going and having a sleep study. I did it. You go...

PEGGY: You mean, everybody should do that?

DR PERLMUTTER: Oh, absolutely.

PEGGY: Everybody should have a sleep study?

DR PERLMUTTER: It's very, very important. You talked about *The Grain Brain Whole Life Plan*, and it's in the book.

PEGGY: Yeah.

DR PERLMUTTER: Why? Because you may be going to sleep at a reasonable hour, waking up at a reasonable hour. You've got your eight to ten hours of sleep thinking, "Well, I'm doing what I can."

But in reality you may be arousing several times during the night, multiple times during the night, and this is really not going to be the restorative type of sleep that your brain needs to clean up, to consolidate memory, and to rid itself of accumulated debris, which happens during sleep – debris that would otherwise compromise brain function.

You may have sleep apnea, where you stop breathing, and ultimately gasp for air, arousing you, taking you out of deep, restorative sleep – but you don't even know it. How will you know?

PEGGY: Your partner might know it.

DR PERLMUTTER: Your partner might know it, or your partner, he or she, may be sleeping through the night and not paying any attention. But this is really important, because, again, you don't know it. Your partner might not know it. Have a sleep study.

PEGGY: Okay, what's the relationship between sleep and BDNF? We've got to bring everything back to BDNF.

DR PERLMUTTER: That's a very interesting relationship, that chronic issues with sleep are related to compromised BDNF, but in the very, very short run – as in one or two nights of sleep deprivation – strangely, BDNF is actually increased. Now, I'm not recommending to increase BDNF by depriving yourself of sleep.

PEGGY: No, no.

DR PERLMUTTER: But it's much like caloric restriction or fasting, that in the short run, a level of stress seems to be good for us.

PEGGY: We're not meant to have life too easy.

DR PERLMUTTER: No, we're not, and it's like weightlifting. Weightlifting – when it's done acutely, when you're at the gym, and you're doing curls, you're tearing fibers, you're breaking down your muscle –what happens is that stress, over the next 36 hours, rebuilds those muscle fibers, and then a little bit more.

That's how weightlifting leads to increased size and strength. It's because it repairs the problem, but then goes one step further.

PEGGY: Right.

DR PERLMUTTER: And it's very similar with fasting, and aerobic exercise, and sleep deprivation. But if you were to do curls for 16 hours your biceps would be destroyed. Similarly, if you were to overdo it on the sleep deprivation, then – same thing – you know, there's a sweet spot.

PEGGY: Right.

DR PERLMUTTER: When you exceed the sweet spot night after night, and you don't even know it, that is profoundly detrimental for the brain, and is associated with increased risk for Alzheimer's. Those individuals who have sleep apnea have a dramatically increased risk for Alzheimer's.

All the things that we've been talking about are looking at what is good for the brain, but also in the background should be this poster of preventing that disease in the first place.

There's nothing really heroic, as a medical doctor, about preventing something from happening in the first place. We, as medical doctors, are called in when there's a problem already, so we can be the heroes and cure the disease, or operate on the patient and fix the problem.

But the reality is that preventing disease makes the best sense, because then it doesn't manifest. It makes the best sense economically, because we're going to be spending less health care dollars on treating people. And the whole notion of health care dollars is really interesting, because, by and large, that has nothing to do with health.

You know, these programs that are created in Washington, and whether it survives or doesn't survive, truthfully, has very little to do with health. It's an illness-based program. How will we take care of people when they develop X, Y or Z, whether acutely, in an emergency situation, or as chronic diseases like heart disease, diabetes, cancer, and Alzheimer's.

What can we do to help these people? I think that's noble, but I think much more important is the notion of keeping people healthy in the first place.

PEGGY: Well, you use the term here that the doctor's the hero, because he rushes in, and...

DR PERLMUTTER: Or she.

PEGGY: Or she, yes. I noticed that. Doctors rush in and cure this dramatic problem, and then you're the hero. But I think you're the hero. I mean, they're heroes too, but I think you're the hero by educating.

You call yourself an empowering neurologist, because you empower us with the knowledge to take care of our own brains. I think that's quite heroic. You've been bringing the public this information that, really, nobody else has. And you've certainly been popularizing it in a way that nobody else has.

DR PERLMUTTER: Well, empowerment happens when we receive knowledge, and that is the mission. Because once you have the knowledge, then you can take action. So have the knowledge, take the action, then reap the benefits. That's the mission.

PEGGY: We're getting towards the end, but I want to bring up something you stress in your book, *The Grain Brain Whole Life Plan*. You stress the importance of gratitude, of approaching life with gratitude as an antidote to stress and to depression, which are correlated, of course, with Alzheimer's. Talk to us about gratitude.

DR PERLMUTTER: Well, I think it's an often-overlooked part of the puzzle here. We talked about stress, and sleep, and supplements, and diet, and physical activity...

PEGGY: Right.

DR PERLMUTTER: Your brain actually changes when you express and act on your feelings of gratitude. Research has demonstrated that. I think that gratitude is the antidote to the detrimental effects of stress.

When we are in conflicting environments, that is stressful. That is really kind of what underlies stress, is when we're in an environment that is conflicting with what would otherwise be peaceful for us. And I think that a surefire way to get out of that situation is to rework your day-to-day mentality to a state of gratitude, and not just being grateful for all that is going on, but acting on it, and giving back.

Now, I'm going to tell you that of all the things we've talked about, this really has probably the least scientific underpinning. I think that will change, but this is one that comes from me as an intuitive recommendation, as opposed to a scientific-based recommendation. Truthfully, scientific research has supported everything we've talked about thus far.

So maybe this is getting away from the science of medicine to the art of medicine, and this now becomes Dr. Permutter speaking from what I feel, rather than what my rational mind has allowed me to put forth.

PEGGY: Understood. When you talk about gratitude, and the importance of gratitude, it's something I think we literally feel in our gut. And you've talked about the importance of the gut, the gut bacteria, the connection to the brain...

We know in our gut if we feel content, if we feel satisfied, if we're in a place of negativity, or if we're in a place of feeling grateful and connected in a positive way in the world. We feel it in our gut. And that's kind of an argument. You said it's not scientific, but it's something I think we intuitively feel physically.

DR PERLMUTTER: I'll tell you an interesting experience that I had recently. We were hiking in Utah, my wife and I. We came upon a sign on the trail, and the sign had an arrow going left, and an arrow going right. And the arrow going left said, "For Climbers," and the arrow going right said, "For Hikers."

PEGGY: Okay.

DR PERLMUTTER: And I could've lamented the fact that I didn't feel comfortable being the climber anymore.

PEGGY: Right.

DR PERLMUTTER: But instead, I was grateful for the fact that I can still be the hiker.

PEGGY: You can still be the hiker, and your wife is with you to hike with you, and you ought to be grateful for that...

DR PERLMUTTER: Right. So it is being grateful for what you can do, not what you can't do. If you can't run the three miles, be grateful for the fact that you can walk out of your front door and get to the mailbox.

It's really embracing and celebrating the glass that's half-full – what you can achieve in this world, what you can do – as opposed to lamenting what no longer is available.

PEGGY: Well, what we can do is do the program that you laid out for us. The responsibility is on us. It's our own brains, and the responsibility is for us to take the knowledge that you've empowered us with, and to make it our own.

Let me just leave you with this question. *The Grain Brain Whole Life Plan* – talk to us about that. It's a plan. How do we get ourselves to plan? We know we have to do this in order to take care of our brains. How do we go about planning brain health...?

DR PERLMUTTER: Well, that's what the plan is all about – what are the things we take? How do we change our diets? Why is sleep so important? What is the importance of gratitude? What about nutritional supplements? What about this whole idea of nurturing our gut bacteria? That's what went into the book.

I wrote a book called *Grain Brain*, and *Grain Brain* focused on carbohydrates and sugar, as well as gluten.

PEGGY: Right.

DR PERLMUTTER: Following that, I wrote *Brain Maker* that focused on the gut bacteria. Those books were much more about the "why." Why is the science telling us what it's telling us? What is it telling us is important?

The new book is really about the "how." Now, how do we leverage that information and create a plan, so that day-to-day we know we are nurturing our health, and specifically, nurturing our brain?

Now I'm going to do something that's really quite unusual for an interview, and that is, I'm going to ask you, now that we've spent this time together, what will change with you as you move forward, having had this interview with me and hearing this information?

PEGGY: Okay, I'll say that after the last interview that we did, I changed, because you'd told me about your breakfast, that it was coffee with coconut oil. And you said you could go till eleven, or noon, or one o'clock, and I thought, "He must be so hungry!"

But I began doing that. I add butter to it, and that's my breakfast, and I can, indeed, go till eleven or noon without eating... So you've already changed me. You know what I'm going to say.

DR PERLMUTTER: I know what you're going to say.

PEGGY: I'm going to exercise. I'm going to put on James Brown.

DR PERLMUTTER: "I Feel Good."

PEGGY: "I Feel Good," and I'm going to dance. That's what I'm going to do.

DR PERLMUTTER: Good.

PEGGY: So I – yes, I promise you. You have my word.

DR PERLMUTTER: Okay. The next interview we do, I'm going to check up on you.

PEGGY: Yeah, you're going to check up...

DR PERLMUTTER: Terrific.

PEGGY: I'll show you my dance moves. Okay. Thank you so much, Dr. Perlmutter.

DR PERLMUTTER: My pleasure, my pleasure, absolutely.

PEGGY: Thank you so much for watching. I hope you learned a lot from Dr. Perlmutter today. A lot of this information is in his book, which is a terrific book, *The Grain Brain Whole Life Plan*, and you'll find more specifics there to reinforce your motivation to do all the brain-friendly things that Dr. Perlmutter described today. Thank you for watching.

Interview with Michael Fossel, M.D., Ph.D.

PEGGY: Hello. I'm Peggy Sarlin, and today I'm in San Rafael, California, with Dr. Michael Fossel, and he's going to tell you a story that I think will astound you.

Dr. Fossel is at the forefront of an Alzheimer's revolution. He's developed a completely new approach that he thinks will reverse, and even outright cure Alzheimer's in people – not just mice – in just a few years.

And not only that – Dr. Fossel believes that the same approach can be used to reverse all diseases of aging, from arthritis, to osteoporosis, to Parkinson's, to macular degeneration – on and on and on.

Now, what Dr. Fossel's going to say may sound a little bit like science fiction to you, so I'm going to take a little more time than I usually do to tell you his background, so you can judge for yourself his credibility. He got his M.D. and Ph.D. at Stanford University, where he taught neurobiology and research methods. He served as Executive Director of the American Aging Association, and was Founding Editor of Rejuvenation Research.

He wrote the definitive textbook on cellular aging, and he's regarded as the world's foremost expert on clinical use of telomerase for age-related diseases. You may have heard of telomeres and telomerase, but you're going to hear a lot more today about their really revolutionary potential for arthritis, Alzheimer's – all age-related diseases.

So this man thinks big. Welcome, Dr. Fossel.

DR MICHAEL FOSSEL: Thank you, Peggy. Pleasure to be here with you.

PEGGY: All right, so the world of Alzheimer's is filled with doom and gloom, and so many failed efforts and dead ends, and you feel exactly the opposite. Tell us, in your view, in view of what you're trying to do, if everything just goes as smoothly as humanly possible, what's the world going to look like in three years?

DR FOSSEL: I think within three years, we can demonstrate that we can both prevent and cure Alzheimer's disease. We should have human trial results by then, so let's see what happens.

PEGGY: So you are preparing now to do human trials on this unique treatment for Alzheimer's.

DR FOSSEL: That's correct.

PEGGY: We're not talking about 10 years, 20 years... We're talking about right now, it's in the works.

DR FOSSEL: And it's interesting you say that, because most of these trials have to be extensive and take years, and have just minimal statistical results. I think we can demonstrate pretty clear results, and do it fairly quickly, too.

PEGGY: I'll go back to that question. What's the world going to look like? What does a cure look like? We haven't heard that word. What does a cure look like for Alzheimer's? What are you going to do to these people, and how are they going to change?

DR FOSSEL: That's a lot of questions!

PEGGY: That's a lot of questions, but you can handle them.

DR FOSSEL: We're pretty confident. What that'll look like is they'll be better. I think it's hard for any of us to believe that you can get a complete reversal of everything, no matter how far down the road you go. But we've been astounded in the animal results with what we can get back.

To put it bluntly, I think we can take people with moderate Alzheimer's and reverse most of the cognitive defect. I think we can bring them back pretty much to normal. That's what we're aiming at.

PEGGY: Now, when I said that your approach is different, your approach does not involve lots of different health prescriptions for the patient, that they must do this, they must do that every day. They must eat this, and take this supplement... No, no, no. Tell us what you're going to do for these people.

DR FOSSEL: Well, let me put it this way: We don't know very many 10-year-olds, or 20-year-olds who have Alzheimer's. We know a lot of people in their 60s and 70s with Alzheimer's. And what we're essentially doing is resetting the cells to act more like younger cells again.

The risks that you had when you were 10 and 20 – which is to say, not many – will be the risks that we'll be able to bring you back to by resetting those cells to act like young cells again.

PEGGY: And to reset the cells, the actual physical treatment is an injection.

DR FOSSEL: It is. And now, in the long run, we think we can deliver it nasally, maybe orally, certainly by IV... there's any number of ways we're going to be able to deliver it. We're going to start by using an injection, sort of like an epidural or subdural would, because it's probably the most reasonable approach to take for a first trial. But ultimately, I think we can make it a lot easier to use, and a lot cheaper.

PEGGY: A whole lot cheaper, if you can take somebody with, as you said, moderate Alzheimer's, which is an extraordinarily expensive condition to treat. You're going to just give them an injection, and they're going to be okay.

DR FOSSEL: Essentially, yes. It's a one-time injection, and what it does is it takes a human gene and instructs the cells to reset their pattern of gene expression so they act more like young cells. They begin to do their job, clean up cellular garbage, in a sense, in a way that young cells do.

Now, my guess is – and it's not just a guess; it's a pretty good prediction – that people will need a repeat treatment in five years or ten years. So it's not permanent, but it's sort of like saying we're going to take your 70-year-old brain, and, as I say, make it a 40- or 50-year-old brain. But then it ages again, and we'll have to reset it later.

PEGGY: So just to recap this, because this is a completely new idea for most people listening, you're starting human trials very soon that you believe will demonstrate, within a period of six months, or a year...

DR FOSSEL: Six months.

PEGGY: ...that you can give a one-time injection, or an injection every five years, and take away Alzheimer's.

DR FOSSEL: I think so. I think we can certainly prevent it, and we can cure much more than we had hoped. Again, I think of it sometimes as a "Humpty Dumpty effect." There've got to be times when the egg shells are broken, and maybe you can't get everything back. There have to be limits.

But the limits are a lot broader than we thought. It looks like we'll be able to take people with fairly moderate advanced Alzheimer's, and get remarkable improvement.

PEGGY: And so to keep the good news going, this is the same principle – which we will get into. We will help our audience understand what this magic injection is, because it sounds like magic.

DR FOSSEL: Well, medical science always sounds like magic when it first gets there.

PEGGY: And this is totally brand new.

This same principle of the injection, when you're dealing with people with Alzheimer's, it's obviously – we hope – going to positively affect their brain, specific areas in the brain. But you believe this same principle can help improve, reverse, cure all diseases of aging... So tell us a little bit about that beautiful picture.

DR FOSSEL: Well, let me start with Alzheimer's since it's our primary strategic first target, and part of the reason is because people don't think you can do anything. And we're pretty sure we can, so we're going to make our point there.

Also, it's a disease that, as you know, is fatal, and we have nothing to treat it with, essentially. So we're going to start with Alzheimer's.

But we're certainly going to move on to the other dementias, whether it's frontal dementia, frontal temporal dementia, Lewy body dementia, or Parkinson's dementia, maybe ALS as well. And after that, we'll be going on to arterial disease.

I mean, most people don't die of Alzheimer's. The most common cause of death for us as we get older is arterial disease – heart attacks, strokes, aneurysms, peripheral vascular disease, congestive heart failure... it goes on and on. And all of those can be traced back to a similar sort of problem to what's going in the brain.

In the brain, we're looking at cells that take care of neurons. They're called "glial cells." And when we're looking at arterial disease, you're looking at the cells that line the blood vessels, for example, in your coronary arteries.

But in every case, what we're doing is resetting the pattern of gene expression to what it used to be, and the cells begin to act like normal, young cells again. So yes, the second big market is arterial disease, followed by things like, as you said, osteoarthritis, osteoporosis, and so forth.

PEGGY: May it all come to pass, because it sounds like a miracle. I want to take people through it step-by-step, so they understand what this treatment is, what the basis of it is. And I thought a good place to start would be with Oprah Winfrey. (See, I like to surprise people, because they didn't think I was going to say that.)

Oprah Winfrey recently made a film called "The Immortal Life of Henrietta Lacks." So tell us, who is Henrietta Lacks? How does her story have relevance to your work?

DR FOSSEL: Well, Henrietta Lacks had a cancer, and the cancer cells were isolated. And one of the things that occurs with many cancer cells, and particularly, what are called "HeLa cells," from Henrietta Lacks...

... is that those cells don't age. Well, they're not the only cells that don't. For example, the cells that created you and me, the ova and sperm, the germ cells for human beings, don't age, either. So some cells age, some don't. Henrietta Lacks' cancer cells don't age. And they were the first cells that we really isolated that were, essentially, immortal cells.

PEGGY: So the principle that the story of Henrietta Lacks establishes... I think I read somewhere that although she's been dead for many years, there's something like tons of cancer cells that have been made from her original cells. They just keep going.

DR FOSSEL: Literally tons.

PEGGY: Literally tons. The cancer cells, by being immortal, they keep dividing, and making more, and more, and more cells.

DR FOSSEL: Right.

PEGGY: So the problem for people with cancer is these are bad guy cells, and yet they have immortal life, and germs, also.

DR FOSSEL: Well, germ cells.

PEGGY: Germ cells.

DR FOSSEL: Ova and sperm are called "germ cells," collectively. You came from a cell you got from your mother with genetic information, and from your father as well. But the cell you got from your mother, she got from your grandmother, who got it from your great-grandmother... That cell went all the way back, didn't age. Your cells age, but the germ cell line goes backwards in time...

So theoretically, I could say you're 3 1/2 billion years old in this planet. You look marvelous for your age.

PEGGY: I do!

DR FOSSEL: You know? But not all cells age. Cancer cells, many don't age. Certain germ cells don't age. Certain other cells, stem cells in your body, age at different rates, depending on how important they are to us.

It's one of the reasons that you and I don't run out of blood cells by the time we're 110. It's because the cells that produce those blood cells age at a very slow rate.

PEGGY: So we've established a principle here that cells age at different rates, and some cells seem to be like the cancer cell – seem to be immortal. So the model in our head isn't that, oh, there's a human body, and it's kind of rusting away, and everything's kind of deteriorating. In fact, no. Different cells are aging at different rates, and...

DR FOSSEL: And when you think about it, we all know this. I mean, those of you who have pets know that your dogs tend to age faster than you and I do. People typically say seven times as fast, but it depends on the dog. Cats may age faster. Mice certainly age faster. You know an average mouse is very old at two years. You and I may be 80 years.

So it's not simply a matter of age, age in terms of years. It's something more than that. Now, that's what you're getting at.

PEGGY: That's what I'm getting at. So the question for – that you ask yourself, if I may presume to...

DR FOSSEL: Is why?

PEGGY: Is why? Why does the cancer cell stay immortal, while other cells, such as cells in the brain, may die?

DR FOSSEL: Age faster, right.

PEGGY: May age, and then eventually die. That's the beginning question that you ask yourself.

DR FOSSEL: Well, it's not even a matter of them dying. My skin cells may not be dead, but they still may have wrinkles. You know, I may still have wrinkles in older skin.

But the cells in your brain are like that, too. The neurons don't age as fast because they don't divide, but the glial cells that take care of the neurons in your brain, those do divide, and as they divide, they age. They change their pattern of gene expression, and they become less and less capable of taking care of the nerve cells. And after while, the nerve cells pay the price of that.

PEGGY: Well, typically, the treatments for Alzheimer's are focused on the nerve cells, right? The nerve cells get covered in plaque. They get these tangles, and we're going to fix the nerve cells, the neurons.

And your approach is very different. You said, "We're going to focus on what surrounds the nerve cells, the glia." Did I get that right...? Okay, you say it in your words.

DR FOSSEL: Well, that's pretty much right.

PEGGY: Okay.

DR FOSSEL: You should say, there are three sorts of approaches to this. One is to ignore the whole problem, and just deal with the way the neurons talk to one another. There are a number of drugs on the market – five on the global market right now – that we use for Alzheimer's, and none of them affect anything except the way neurons talk to each other. But they don't affect the fact that the neurons are dying.

Now, in the past decade or two, most big pharmaceutical companies and little biotech companies have gone upstream a bit, and they've said, "Let's look at beta-amyloid," and as you've said, tau tangles. And there are literally dozens and dozens of other things at that level that they focused on.

But our approach – actually, for the last 20 years, but now we're beginning to come to the human trials – has been to say, "Why are all of these things going wrong at once – beta-amyloid, tau tangles, mitochondria – all of these things? What's going on upstream?"

And over the past, maybe decade, more and more people have begun to realize something's going on with glial cells. Well, we know why something's going wrong. As I say, they're changing their pattern of gene expression. It's not that the glial cell is sick or dead. It's not. It's just not playing the same tune. It's not doing its job as rapidly, so it's not taking care of the neurons.

The beta-amyloid should be taken care of, the tau tangles, and all the other things that affect neurons. So the outcome is Alzheimer's, but the cause is not beta-amyloid. It's upstream.

PEGGY: Just to help us understand the anatomy of the brain: You've got a neuron. You've got a cell, and it's surrounded? These are like guardians, these...? Most of us don't know the term "glia," a glial cell. That's a new concept for us.

DR FOSSEL: We used to say that only one in 10 cells in your brain were actually neurons, and the rest were glia. And it turns out it's not quite that big of a number. Glial cells may be as few as one-to-one, the ratio of glia to neurons, or even two-to-one, but not a huge number. But they're critical.

The glial cells, think of them as the nursing care, the devoted spouse, the staff, the aides... They're the ones who take care of the neurons, wait on them hand and foot. And without those glial cells, the neurons can't function – and they don't.

PEGGY: So when they wait on the neuron, hand and foot... when they give them this tender loving care...

DR FOSSEL: They do.

PEGGY: That's cleaning out toxic waste that might accumulate. What are some of the tasks they're performing to keep that neuron healthy?

DR FOSSEL: Well, I'll give you an example. You know, beta-amyloid has been something we've known about for decades now. Alzheimer's was described 110 years ago this year. But we've known about beta-amyloid for many decades.

But beta-amyloid doesn't just sit there throughout your life. It's continually being turned over. It's dynamic. It's being recycled, and the recycling rate slows with the age of the glial cell.

So in a young person, if you take a 20-year-old, their glial cells are producing beta-amyloid, then they grab onto it. They bring it inside. They break it down, and they make more. And they grab it, bring it inside, break it down, and make more.

But in an older brain, the glial cells are slowing down. So the turnover rate is slower, and as a result the beta-amyloid sits out there longer, and has more time to accumulate damage. It's not being taken in and fixed as quickly.

So overall, it's as though I were to say, "I've got a house, and I can either repaint my walls and fix my carpets once every 50 years, or I can do it once a week." Well, there'll be a dramatic difference in what the house looks like, and weekly maintenance would cost too much.

But you know what I mean. If I only paint my house every few decades, it begins to go downhill. If I paint it every year, it's gonna look like a million dollars.

That's kind of the difference that's going on in the brain cells. Young cells are repainting all the time. Old cells – "Ah, I'll get to it someday."

PEGGY: So you're looking at the glia cells. These are, let's say, the housekeepers, providing the tender, loving care. They're slowing down, and you're saying, "Well, if the cancer cell can be so active, and energetic, and immortal, can I make the glia cells start acting...?"

The cancer cell's the bad guy cell. The glia cell's the good guy cell. Can I get the glia cell, the good guy cell, to be active, and energetic, and immortal, and energetic, like the bad guy cell? Is that kind of the starting question you ask yourself?

DR FOSSEL: Kind of, yes. No cells are really immortal. It's a question of do they continue to divide forever if you keep giving them food, as it were,?

PEGGY: Immortal.

DR FOSSEL: Immortal. As I say, you know, the human race is immortal in some sense. We've been around a long time. We don't age as a race, but we age as individuals.

But the cells are the same way. We're not making those cells immortal, but we're bringing them back to the same stage they were when you were younger. So again, they will age again, but we can reset them again to a pattern of gene expression.

It's as though you had a symphony orchestra – and that's the genes – and the difference is, the older cells are playing a totally different tune, you know? One symphony orchestra is playing Mozart, and the other is playing The Grateful Dead – depending which one you like the best.

But you can reset the script. You can reset the score they're playing. It's not a problem with the instruments. It's not that as you get older, the genes don't work. They're just playing a different tune.

And what we do is say, "You know what? Play the score you were playing when you were working well." And they do.

It's as though you're at a house... how fast do I vacuum it, or how fast do I clean the kitchen? Well, if you do it once a month, the house looks bad. If you vacuum your house once a week, it looks better. We're saying, "Reset the cleaning schedule, please. Pick up the maintenance."

PEGGY: So it's not immortality, but it's resetting the clock. It's all our dream, turning back the clocks of time.

DR FOSSEL: Oddly enough, we first did this, now, 18 years ago, with human cells. It was the first time with human tissues, 17 years ago, and a whole set of them about that same time. But we're getting to the point now where we're able to do this with whole animals – mice, people. So it's an exciting time.

PEGGY: This is a very new science, and you're saying it was 17, 18 years ago that this principle was established, that it could be done, that the reset could be done.

DR FOSSEL: If 20 years is new, yes.

PEGGY: So all right, now I think it's time we start letting people know how you do this magic – it feels like magic – and it involves the use of telomeres, which is kind of a new word in the public eye, I think. People may have heard that word, telomeres, and not know exactly what they are. Tell us about telomeres, and how they impact your work.

DR FOSSEL: Well, I think of telomeres, in some sense, as the conductor of that symphony orchestra. The telomeres are the piece at the end of each chromosome. And frankly, the telomeres themselves don't matter, and the length of the telomere doesn't matter. What matters is that, as the length changes, they change the pattern of gene expression throughout the rest of your cells. That's critical.

So, you know, telomeres aren't the cause of aging. They're just one piece in the puzzle. The key question for me is, can we understand enough of what's going on there that we can fix it? And the really critical question is, what's the most effective place to intervene to fix these things?

The telomere is that most effective place, but by itself, the telomere is just part of a big cascade of things going on in aging cells.

PEGGY: So we have our goal. Our goal is that we're going to reset the clock of the glial cells, the glial cells that surround the neuron, and that keep it nice, and freshly vacuumed, and dusted...

DR FOSSEL: The goal is to save lives, or save minds.

PEGGY: Okay, the technique.

DR FOSSEL: But you're right, you're right.

PEGGY: Okay. We have our technique. We have our clinical goal, which is, we're aiming at resetting the clock of the glial cells so that they're going to be nice, tidy, active, efficient housekeepers once again for our precious neuron cells.

DR FOSSEL: Right. That's it.

PEGGY: And somehow, somehow – and you're going to help us understand – somehow, the telomeres of the glia cells are going to be the key to doing this.

DR FOSSEL: That's a nice, quick way to put it, but yes, they take care of most of the problems that happen with neurons. The neuron itself is sort of the innocent bystander. The glial cells are doing their best to take care of things, but again, as they get older, they change their rate of maintenance, and the neurons are the ones that pay for it.

They pay for it in terms of beta-amyloid plaque, and tau tangles, as you mentioned, and they die. And the outcome is that you and I lose our minds.

PEGGY: So the job of the telomere is to, in some way, control the efficiency of the glia cell?

DR FOSSEL: Sets the pace.

PEGGY: It sets the pace.

DR FOSSEL: It sets the pace of maintenance for the rest of that cell. So for example, look at DNA repair. All of us know that your risk of cancer goes up with age, and it goes up exponentially. But if I ask myself why that is, it turns out that the DNA repair enzymes in your cells – again, the rate of that repair is controlled by the telomere. And as our cells gets older, the rate slows down, so you're no longer as capable of repairing little mutations.

Now, in just talking in the last few minutes, every one of our cells has probably had a mutation, and probably within milliseconds, it's been repaired. But that delay, the time it takes to make the repair, gets slower and slower as we get older. And it's the telomere that sets the pace of that repair.

You still repair. You just don't do it as quickly, so you're a little more likely to accumulate damage as you get older. Hence, cancer, Alzheimer's, arterial disease... they all tend to come back to this same common denominator, gene expression, telomeres, cell aging.

PEGGY: So let's go back to Henrietta Lacks, and the cancer cells. Her cancer cell is staying vigorous and efficient over time, as opposed to the glia cell in the human brain that's winding down, that's getting less efficient. What is different about the telomere in the cancer cell, as opposed to the telomere in the glia cell?

DR FOSSEL: Well, let me distinguish three different kinds of cells. First, we'll take the germ cell line – the ova, the sperm that create human beings. Those cells maintain their telomeres all the time. They keep a good, long telomere. They're always efficient.

At the other extreme, we have most of our body cells in which the telomeres are shortened with age, and so the pattern of cell maintenance goes down, and down, and down.

The cancer cells lie sort of in between that, in a sense, because they maintain their telomeres. They don't shorten very much, but they're not very long in the first place.

So the problem is that while they maintain just enough telomere so the cells can divide, they don't maintain enough telomere, for example, to maintain the cell all that well, so it's more prone to cancer. Hence, cancer cells in general.

So Henrietta Lacks' cancer cells maintain their telomeres, but they already have inherited a lot of damage. In fact, they sometimes say that Henrietta Lacks' cells are not really human. They're partly human, partly viral, partly mutation. They're special. But cancer cells in general maintain just enough telomere length to keep dividing, but not enough to fully repair things.

PEGGY: You mentioned telomere length, telomere shortening... I think if people have heard about telomeres, they may be familiar with that concept that the telomere length is important, and as they get shorter, it's less good.

When I discussed your upcoming interview with somebody, they said, "Oh, I just had my telomere length measured, and it's really good." So tell us a little bit about that, because people may have heard about that.

DR FOSSEL: Well, let me first say something that is kind of odd, which is to say, telomere length doesn't matter at all. It's the change in length.

PEGGY: It doesn't matter what you start with; it matters how it changes over time.

DR FOSSEL: I'll give you an example. You know, the average mouse has a lifespan about 40 times less than ours, but its telomere length, in some cases, is as much as, say, 15, 10 to15 times what ours are. So most mice have longer telomeres than you and I do, and yet, we live longer than most mice do.

And the same thing's true here. It's not the length of the telomere that matters; it's the change in length, and how it changes gene expression. So in a mouse, the telomere changes length, changes gene expression. The mouse gets old faster.

With you and I, that change in length goes down a little bit, but we start with a short telomere. But it's that change in length. It's that sort of percentage of change that makes all the difference. It's the gene expression that really makes the difference.

So one common misconception is that telomere length matters. No, it's the change in length that matters, whether you're a mouse, a human, or anything else. Another is that telomeres come apart and fray, like shoelaces. Well, they don't, actually. It's the change in length that makes all the difference in the world.

PEGGY: So just staying with that for a minute, the change in length... every time a cell divides, the telomere slightly shortens.

DR FOSSEL: Right, unless the cell has a way of keeping it long. Now, as I said, germ cells, sperm and ova, keep their telomere lengths. How do they do that?

PEGGY: How do they do that?

DR FOSSEL: They shorten also, but they have an enzyme called telomerase, okay? And what that does, every time the telomere shortens, is it relengthens it slightly. Germ cells have telomerase. Cancer cells, most of them, have just enough telomerase to keep a short telomere from going all the way to zero.

Most of your body's cells don't express telomerase. There are a few special ones, for example, stem cells in your bone marrow express just enough telomerase to keep the telomeres from shortening too much.

But most of your body's cells don't express any telomerase, so every time they divide, they shorten... and every time they shorten, it changes gene expression... and every time that happens, they get less effective at taking care of the cells around them, and themselves.

PEGGY: All right, so you mentioned telomerase, and that's going to be a new word for a lot of people. So I'd like to show everybody your book, *The Telomerase Revolution*. It's a little hard to pronounce. I was pronouncing it differently, but *Telomerase Revolution*. And everything we're talking about today with Dr. Fossel comes down to this, telomerase. So let's understand a little bit more about what it is. Telomerase is an enzyme that is created by telomeres.

DR FOSSEL: No, actually.

PEGGY: No. I'm all wrong. Correct me. Okay, good. That's what you're here for.

DR FOSSEL: Telomerase is an enzyme that relengthens telomeres, but you have a gene –

PEGGY: Wait, no – I didn't hear that. Say it again.

DR FOSSEL: Telomerase is an enzyme that relengthens telomeres.

PEGGY: That relengthens them.

DR FOSSEL: Right. And you have a gene that makes telomerase. But in almost all of your cells, it's turned off. It's like you have a blueprint, but it's locked up.

Now, what we do with our treatment is we put that same blueprint into the cell and say, "Make this, please." And when it does that, it relengthens telomeres, and that resets gene expression, and cells begin to act normally again.

PEGGY: So this is not a question of restoring something that was there before. They never had telomerase. You're introducing something new. It's not a question of...

DR FOSSEL: Well, it's a natural human gene. All of your cells have the blueprint. It's just usually not expressed. They don't make it.

PEGGY: Right.

DR FOSSEL: And we're just saying, "Here's another blueprint. Make this one. The one you have that's locked up? Make this one." It's the same natural gene. We all have it. It's a human gene.

PEGGY: So the cancer cell is expressing telomerase...

DR FOSSEL: A little bit.

PEGGY: ...and now you're going to get the glia cells to express telomerase.

DR FOSSEL: Just enough to reset the length of the telomere, so a cell begins to act like young cells, like a young glial cell – just enough to do that.

PEGGY: How much is just enough...? You say you're going to give an injection. How much telomerase is going to make this miracle last for five years? Is it like this much?

DR FOSSEL: Oh, it's much less than the end of your thumb. It's a tiny amount.

PEGGY: Less – we're just going to have that much?

DR FOSSEL: Oh, even less. We give it in a small syringe. It's a tiny amount. Just enough. That's all it takes.

PEGGY: I said this sounds like science fiction, and it does. You're going to get this tiny injection, and how does it know where to go?

DR FOSSEL: Yes, there are two parts to this. It's like having an envelope and a letter, and we have an envelope. It's a biological envelope that we've got, and we change the address. So the address on it says, "Please go to the glial cells."

And inside there's a letter and what we've done is put in our own letter, and it says, "Please make normal human telomerase gene." We put the letter in the envelope, and we inject it into you, and it's addressed to your cells, so it knows where to go.

Your cells look at the letter and say, "This is meant for me." So they bring it inside. They open it up, look at the letter, and it says, "Make telomerase," and they say, "Done." Now, as you might guess, it's more complicated than that.

PEGGY: Yes.

DR FOSSEL: But I think that's a good analogy.

PEGGY: Since you're starting with Alzheimer's, that's your first target. So when you give this injection of telomerase (I'll get used to that pronunciation)...

DR FOSSEL: Any pronunciation is fine. They're all right. None of us have accents. Everyone else does. Right.

PEGGY: You have designed this to say, "Go to the glial cells in the brain." But you could design it differently to say, for example, "Go to the arthritic joints."

DR FOSSEL: Correct. Or the coronary arteries.

PEGGY: Or the retina of the eye, or the...

DR FOSSEL: Any of the above.

PEGGY: Tell us some of the diseases that you see using the same very simple injection with the specifically-designed envelope, designed to deliver telomerase to those cells. You mentioned coronary disease as your next project. You're starting with neurodegenerative diseases.

DR FOSSEL: Well, let me give you an example of this. If I just adjust the glial cells, I can probably not only go after Alzheimer's, but Parkinson's.

Now, everyone knows – I mean, I know, having taught this for years – Alzheimer's patients tend to make certain things, like beta amyloid plaque, and tau tangles.

PEGGY: Right.

DR FOSSEL: And Parkinson's patients tend to make a different kind of a problem called Alpha-synuclein. But never mind the technicality. The question is, why are they all making these things? And upstream, it's the same problem.

In parts of the brain, if the glial cells don't work right, I've got the Parkinson's problem, and in other parts of the brain, if the glial cells aren't working right, I've got beta-amyloid, and I've got Alzheimer's disease.

So the upstream problem is the same. It's sort of expressed different ways. Parkinson's, Alzheimer's, other forms of dementia.

Now, if you look at things like vascular dementia, another form of dementia, it's because of the blood supply to parts of the brain, and there, you're looking at the cells that line the vessels. They're called "endothelial cells."

We've known now for 17 years that we can take old human endothelial cells, reset the telomeres, and grow what looks like young human arterial tissue. The trick is being able to do that in patients to save lives. And that's where we have finally gotten in just the last few years.

PEGGY: It's so exciting. Alzheimer's starts in the hippocampus, as most people who are watching this probably know, because they're interested. So this injection would go, as the envelope says, "to the hippocampus, to the glial cells." They open it up, and it says, "Okay, hippocampal glial cells, start making an enzyme called telomerase."

DR FOSSEL: Correct, right.

PEGGY: For Parkinson's...

DR FOSSEL: Again, it's wildly more technically difficult than that, but...

PEGGY: Yeah!

DR FOSSEL: But in a sense, that hits it right on the head. You hit it, Peggy.

PEGGY: Okay, okay. Parkinson's disease involves a different part of the brain – what's the part of the brain where Parkinson's is located?

DR FOSSEL: Well, you're usually looking at a place called the *substantia nigra*, but it's not – again, it's never quite that simple. For example, we know that Parkinson's disease patients will sometimes have cognitive problems like Alzheimer's.

PEGGY: Right.

DR FOSSEL: And Alzheimer's patients will sometimes have motor problems like Parkinson's. So there's an overlap, in some sense, and that's in a way the first clue that there's more going on that they share upstream, the glial cell dysfunction.

So when we are sending this in, we're sending it in to all the glial cells. It will go for these ones; it'll go for these ones. Our first target is Alzheimer's disease, but the reason is pretty simple. If I go out now to my neurologist and say, "I've got Parkinson's disease," there are lots of trials out there. Some of them have some effect. There are drugs that we've had around now for decades. I've been using for decades, L-dopa comes to mind. It's been around a long time.

But there's really nothing that's had any effect on Alzheimer's disease, so that's really our primary target, but it's the same target for both, and for all the other dementias I can think of except vascular dementia, where we're not dealing with the glial cells but with blood vessels.

But again, the general approach – resetting cell aging – is effective in human tissue, and human cells, human tissues, and in animals. So it's trying to take it to patient care.

PEGGY: So Doctor, you've told us all these diseases of aging that might ultimately be improved, or even cured, by the same simple injection that directly targets the relevant glia cells.

DR FOSSEL: Sounds simple.

PEGGY: Sounds simple. I'm not saying what you're doing is simple.

DR FOSSEL: It's hard.

PEGGY: Don't misinterpret me.

DR FOSSEL: Right.

PEGGY: I'm trying to make it simple for the audience to understand, not simple to actually execute. But what can't this do? What medical problems can this approach not do?

DR FOSSEL: Oh, a million things. You know, if you're dealing with diseases that are associated with aging, it can probably prevent and cure potentially all of them. But we don't just die of age-related diseases. We die of trauma, sometimes self-inflicted. We die of infectious diseases. Ebola comes to mind. Influenza... There are endless diseases. There are genetic diseases that people are born with. All sorts of things that happen, and this affects almost none of them.

PEGGY: Okay, so it's not a get out of jail free pass. The other doctors that I speak to – I speak to many doctors on these topics – put the emphasis on lifestyle.

The emphasis is you're going to eat in a certain brain-healthy way. You're going to exercise in a brain-healthy way. You're going to sleep...your whole life is going to be on a path of brain-healthy living. And you're saying, "Oh, I'll just give you an injection, and you're good to go."

DR FOSSEL: You know, not quite, for two reasons.

One is, what about me? What about now? What about not three years from now, but this year? What do I do? And their approach is right.

The question is, what can I do now? And as I sometimes say, part of what you can do is listen to what your doctor told you. Listen to what your grandmother told you, and it's often the same advice. You probably didn't pay attention to either one, but at least your grandmother's cheaper.

There's a certain amount of innate knowledge that's not sexy: eating right, exercising, taking care of your body in many ways. That advice doesn't change.

But what happens when we begin to treat things like Alzheimer's and coronary artery disease? For example, what happens to you, right now, if you don't exercise and have a horrible diet – you know that you're more likely to get a heart attack, okay? But what if we can prevent that and cure that? Does that mean, as you say, get out of jail free?

No. What it means is maybe now you have the same risk you had when you were 40 years old, rather than when you're 60 years old. But you had some risk when you were 40 also. I've seen 25-year-olds die of heart attacks. Well, I can't make anyone's heart much younger than a 25-year-old.

No, I think we still need to have some sense, some little bit of listening to that grandmother, as it were, or your family doctor. But we can do an awful lot.

PEGGY: I certainly hope so. For people who are hearing this... you're going to be starting the human trials soon, and hopefully, everything will be as smooth, and efficient, and successful way as possible. But it's not something we can do for ourselves today. Is there anything on the market today that we can do to start helping our telomeres?

DR FOSSEL: You remember I said that the first time we ever reversed aging human cells was now 18 years ago, in 1999, and then followed by some human tissues experiments shortly thereafter. The question is, have we ever done any experiments on human beings, showing that we can do something with telomerase?

The answer is, actually, yes. I know there have been at least three or four papers published looking at telomerase activators, as they're called, often abbreviated TA. And there's a drug on the market, TA-65, for example, but there are other similar agents out there that are supposed to be the same thing.

Well, we know that these agents, if they are honestly what they're supposed to be, can reverse some of the shrinking of telomeres. It's not that they stop it, or reset it totally. But they certainly can slow it slightly. The evidence is fairly good. It doesn't hit you over the head. Nobody has gone from age 70 back to age 30.

But if we look at indications like their bone marrow density, or the way their immune system functions, what you see is fairly good evidence that there's been some improvement, and that's remarkable by itself. Again, we see these telomerase activators work in the lab with human cells and tissues. We see evidence that they work in patients. They're not a panacea, but that's about all there is right now that's out there on the market.

PEGGY: You called it a drug, TA–65. Is it a prescription drug? How do we get this?

DR FOSSEL: No, technically right now it's classified as a nutraceutical, and the reason is that it's actually derived from a root. That root has been used as an herbal tea historically for thousands of years.

So you're dealing with something that's a known quantity, in some sense. It's a known herbal medicine. Well, it's not quite. It's an extract from that. But from a legal perspective, it doesn't qualify as a pharmaceutical. It qualifies as a nutraceutical, so the regulatory constraints are very different.

PEGGY: So you can go to a health food store or you can buy it online.

DR FOSSEL: You can, but are you really getting that? And that's a good question. There are three questions, really. One is, if you go to get these astragalusides, or telomerase activators, are you getting what you pay for?

Second question is, do they really work? I've just told you that there's some evidence they do. There is some evidence. Does that mean they work or not? There is some evidence.

The third one is, is it worth it to you? It depends on how much they cost. Often, they may cost several hundred dollars a month, depending where you get them and how reliable they are. Is that worth it?

Well, that's like saying, "Is my insurance policy worth it?" It depends what they're offering for the policy, and how much money. If I'm on a fixed income with very little, and I'm feeling healthy, then probably not. If I were rich and worried about these age-related diseases, I would take a very different tack on this. But I can't answer that question for anybody.

PEGGY: You mentioned a specific brand called TA–65.

DR FOSSEL: Yeah, TA–65 has been put out by a company called TA Sciences, and they bought the original patent rights to this telomerase activator back now, oh, about 15 years ago. They're probably a reliable source, probably the most reliable source. But there are other sources out there, it's just not clear to many of us whether those other sources are reliable or not.

PEGGY: Okay, but for people who are intrigued by what you've had to say today, and are interested in being good to their telomeres, encouraging the reset of them through telomerase, they can buy TA–65 and other products that are on the market, and decide for themselves whether the price is worth it.

What about Vitamin E? Is that something that is going to positively affect telomere length, or not?

DR FOSSEL: Probably not.

PEGGY: Probably not.

DR FOSSEL: I mean, we start by saying that all of us should have reasonably good diets, and there's been extensive literature now for several decades that we use to deal with at the Aging Association about Vitamin E tocopherols. This sort of comes in and out of fashion, in some sense.

But it is clear that you have a need for it, and it's clear that you need a certain amount at least. You shouldn't be not taking it in a good diet. But what about extra amounts? And the answer probably is, you don't need that.

There's an old joke among pharmacologists that Americans have the most expensive urine in the world, because we buy all these things, and we don't really need them, and we urinate them out.

But it's still a good question, you know? What should we do? What can we do? And there's been a lot of literature in the last couple of years now, looking at what happens to telomere lengths. When I do things like give Vitamin E, or have people get better diet and exercise, or they meditate, the problem is that almost all the literature on these recommendations may be true, but it's not actually well-founded. The problem is they're looking at telomere lengths in my blood cells, and there are several technical problems in that.

So when somebody says, "I've got an article that shows I can increase my telomere lengths by doing the following: exercise, meditation, lowering stress – whatever it is," that may be true, but the evidence actually doesn't support that because of the way these measurements are done.

PEGGY: So we're really rooting for you here, because we want to know that we can just get that simple injection and we're good to go for five years, and all these horrible problems of aging are just going to almost evaporate, if we could look at it that way...

DR FOSSEL: I think so.

PEGGY: In your book, you end with a section that was absolutely fascinating. What is the world going to be like? You are envisioning the possibility of actually doubling the human lifespan. This would keep getting reset. We would reset our cellular age.

DR FOSSEL: No one knows. You know, the mean lifespan worldwide now, depending on the country you're in, runs around 70, 75. The maximum has changed over the last few centuries. It's gone up. The maximum lifespan, the maximum human lifespan, is estimated at around 120.

PEGGY: Right.

DR FOSSEL: So we've got a couple of people who've made that. And that probably has never changed in thousands and thousands of years. More and more people get there, but still not very many.

But that's the kind of lifespan we're looking at altering – not just the mean lifespan, not just that you have a little chance to make it to old age, but you have a good chance of pushing old age back a ways.

So it's a very different approach to human medicine, and what we can do for not only human beings medically, but culturally.

PEGGY: Well, in the book you extrapolate on that idea, the societal changes that result if people are living longer, and you pose some questions. My favorite one was, can marriage last? Can a marriage last 300 years?

DR FOSSEL: Can it last three years?

PEGGY: It can feel like 300 years in certain marriages. That's a good question.

DR FOSSEL: And this doesn't make that better or worse. The problem of getting along with other human beings has been with us for a long time, and this isn't going to change anything.

PEGGY: No, our healthy glial cells are not going to change how we get along, but...

DR FOSSEL: But it will change some things. If I look back and I ask myself, "What are the most important things that happened in medicine in the last few centuries?" They're not the big things. It's not the things that would win a Nobel prize. It's not heart transplants, and it's not a robotic surgery.

If you ask what really changed lives, it was things like Semmelweis, back 150 years ago, saying, "You know, you should wash your hands before and after a delivery"... and Lister saying, "You know, we ought to have antiseptic surgery"... and Pasteur and Koch saying, "You know, maybe germs cause disease, and we could have immunizations"... and then along came our earliest antibiotics with Fleming last century, things like polio vaccines.

These are the things that really made people's lives better, but they also had an impact culturally. I think that what we're about to have is potentially the biggest impact we've ever had on improving people's lives, and that would have cultural impacts as well.

We all get used to the idea that as you approach your 60s and into your 70s, you'll retire, and you'll be too tired to go out dancing Saturday night. Well, some people aren't. Many people may not be. We may find that, in fact, we're a lot healthier. And really, one, you can't afford to retire if you're going to live to 110 and be healthy...

PEGGY: No.

DR FOSSEL: ...and two, why would you want to? Do you really want to do nothing for 40 years? No, I think it's going to change the way we interact as well, but it doesn't make us better people. It just changes the ground rules a little bit.

PEGGY: I started out by saying that you think big, and even saying that underestimates how you think.

DR FOSSEL: Well, let me also say that most of the medical advances that we think of as real advances – as I say, the robotic surgeries and the heart transplants – are expensive. The treatment I'm working on is expensive to get started, but actually, the best projections we've got are that it will lower the global cost of healthcare by an order of 95%.

We're looking at something sort of unheard of in modern health economics. We're looking at actually cutting costs of healthcare. It's a different world.

PEGGY: Well, returning it specifically to Alzheimer's, which is where you're beginning this, that is an extraordinarily expensive disease to treat over time – or not even treat, but just to manage – to care for these people.

DR FOSSEL: And that's only if you look as economically, as opposed to the human cost. But yes.

PEGGY: Yes. But since you mentioned cutting the cost of that, if we did not have to care for people with that disease for ten years... if we could just give them that nice little shot, they're good to go for five years... financially, would that not be an extraordinary achievement, just on that level?

DR FOSSEL: Right now, without any technical advances, my best estimate in doing this is that the cost of treating one person to prevent or cure Alzheimer's disease is about 20% of what it costs to care for an Alzheimer's patient for one year.

PEGGY: For one year. For one year.

DR FOSSEL: And of course, people usually live for years with Alzheimer's, the average is eight years. That's a lot of money, and I'm just talking about needing this treatment once out of every ten years. So yes, I think we can lower costs dramatically.

PEGGY: As I said, you think big, so I want to thank you so much for coming today, and I want to thank you for your work, and wish you all the best for all of our sakes.

DR FOSSEL: Well, thank you for the good wishes, and I hope it succeeds, Peggy.

PEGGY: May it succeed.

DR FOSSEL: Please.

PEGGY: May it blossom. May it help us all.

Thank you so much for watching, and I hope you learned a lot today about this whole exciting, new field of curing age-related diseases through telomerase. What an exciting concept! So maybe I'll see you in 40 years, 50 years. We'll still all be young and vigorous, and have fabulously efficient glial cells, thanks to the work of Dr. Fossel.